The Fertility Promise: The Facts Behind *in vitro* Fertilisation (IVF)

Authored by

Peter Hollands

Freelance Consultant Clinical Scientist
Huntingdon, Cambs, PE26 1LB
UK

The Fertility Promise: The Facts Behind *in vitro* Fertilisation (IVF)

Author: Peter Hollands

ISBN (Online): 978-981-5040-28-9

ISBN (Print): 978-981-5040-29-6

ISBN (Paperback): 978-981-5040-30-2

need for a court order if at any point you breach any terms of this License Agreement. In no event will any delay or failure by Bentham Science Publishers in enforcing your compliance with this License Agreement constitute a waiver of any of its rights.

3. You acknowledge that you have read this License Agreement, and agree to be bound by its terms and conditions. To the extent that any other terms and conditions presented on any website of Bentham Science Publishers conflict with, or are inconsistent with, the terms and conditions set out in this License Agreement, you acknowledge that the terms and conditions set out in this License Agreement shall prevail.

Bentham Science Publishers Pte. Ltd.
80 Robinson Road #02-00
Singapore 068898
Singapore
Email: subscriptions@benthamscience.net

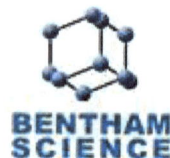

BENTHAM SCIENCE

CONTENTS

PREFACE

My inspiration to write The Fertility Promise has been my experience in assisted reproduction (or IVF) since it was first introduced to me at Bourn Hall Clinic in the early 1980's. I was lucky enough to be one of the first Clinical Embryologists in the world. I have seen IVF move from the initial ideas of Bob Edwards, Patrick Steptoe and Jean Purdy, being carried out in a little village in rural Cambridgeshire, to a billion-Dollar (or Pound!) industry being delivered on a global scale. Many things have changed in IVF during that time. IVF technology has moved on to a certain extent (but with no tangible benefit to patients but with definite financial benefits to clinics and manufacturers) and regulation to ensure optimum quality and safety of all fertility treatments is now routine in most countries. Regulation is extremely important in an area such as IVF to protect both patient and societal safety. Patient expectations, in terms of what a fertility clinic can deliver, have undergone an exponential rise. Unfortunately, the technology in IVF and the people working in IVF have not really met these expectations. Without a change in mind-set these patient expectations will never be met.

IVF has, in my opinion, stagnated in the past 25 years to the point where great change is needed to make further progress and improve the service provided to patients. There have been few effective innovations or new ideas and the live birth rate (which, by the way, is the *only* thing which really matters to all fertility patients) has not really changed since 1978. There are IVF clinics whose sole purpose is to maximise financial profit. There is little or no thought for the well-being of the patients involved or for their hopes, wishes and fears. There are some IVF clinics who deliberately mislead patients to ensure that their profit goals are met. This is not how medicine should be practised and is a very sad reflection on the current practice of IVF.

All physicians and healthcare professionals, in any speciality, have a duty of care to their patients which means that everything which is done to, or for, the patient is in the best interest of the patient. This is sadly not the case in the medical speciality of IVF which is a very sad and depressing reflection on the legacy which was left to us by Bob Edwards, Patrick Steptoe and Jean Purdy. It also means that fertility patients are not getting the care they deserve and need. This is a scandal on a global scale for which everyone involved in these poor practices should be ashamed.

In general terms, the highly vulnerable fertility patient will do anything to make their treatment a success. This is no different to any patient with any sort of problem but over the years I have seen this to be more pronounced in fertility patients. If I told a fertility patient to stand on her head for one hour every day and this will increase her chance of becoming pregnant then I am sure that this patient would do this. If I did this, I would be a very questionable healthcare professional because there is, of course, no evidence that standing on the head will improve fertility treatment outcome and it is therefore not in the best interests of the patient. The combination of vulnerable patients and corporate (sometimes even personal) greed leads us to the present situation in fertility treatment around the globe. There is hype, false promises, deliberately misleading information, false hope, false advice, false science and sometimes even deliberately false claims and marketing. This is destroying the reputation of IVF and seriously inhibiting those who seek to improve the technology with a true focus on patient care.

This book addresses all of these issues using clear, truthful, experienced and unbiased language so that fertility patients can see the true state of IVF. It is not easy reading. You may find some of it shocking. You may find some of it unbelievable but please remember that I only describe what I have seen and know. I have no hidden agenda; my only agenda is to make fertility treatment better for patients. We can repair the damage which has been done to IVF and move forward in an ethical, truthful and professional way. In order to make these changes it will need co-operation from IVF clinics, the IVF equipment and reagent manufacturers, manufacturers of IVF related medication, the IVF regulators and anyone with a financial interest in IVF. These financial interests are often investors or financial giants with a clear vested interest in a fertility clinic or a group of fertility clinics. This is not intrinsically bad until financial interests overtake patient care, then we have a big problem. Staff who work in fertility treatments may well have to change the way in which they currently think to achieve progress. This means *everyone* in the clinic because if these changes in mind-set are not agreed upon across the clinic, then they will be ineffective. It will also need a clear understanding and critical analysis of IVF by fertility patients. This is a big challenge for fertility patients, because at present, it is very difficult for them to see who to trust. IVF patients need to move from being passive victims to becoming active, well informed people who have the knowledge and courage to challenge or question the activity or promises of their IVF clinic. If this book stimulates further debate and ultimate change, then it will be a success and IVF will become a trusted medical treatment once more. This is what I truly want to see, but at present, this is not where we are heading. We are heading towards more lies and profiteering in the name of IVF. The purpose for which IVF was invented, to give the opportunity of having a baby to infertile patients and not to generate excessive profit, will prosper. If not, IVF will continue to stagnate, patients will continue to be tricked and misled, and profits will continue to rise. I make no apologies for some of the hard truth and criticism of IVF in this book. I believe that the time is right for change and this book is the beginning.

CONSENT FOR PUBLICATION

Not applicable.

CONFLICT OF INTEREST

The authors declare no conflict of interest, financial or otherwise.

ACKNOWLEDGEMENTS

Declared none.

Peter Hollands
Freelance Consultant Clinical Scientist
Cambridge, UK

DEDICATION

This book is dedicated to my partner Louise Barrett for her love, dedication and support. I must also thank my cardiac surgeon, Mr Ian Wilson and everyone at Liverpool Heart and Chest Hospital without whom none of this would be possible!.

CHAPTER 1

A Bit of History

Peter Hollands

(An Overview of the Historical Development of IVF from 1978 to the Present Day)

History will be kind to me for I intend to write it.
Winston. S. Churchill

Summary: This chapter introduces the basic history of IVF and fertility treatment and sets the scene for the detailed information presented later in this book. It provides an initial overview of IVF technology from the first birth in 1978 to today and the alternatives to fertility treatment such as adoption. It also considers the growing population of Earth and the possible stagnation of fertility services.

A CHILD IS BORN

On July 25th, 1978, a baby girl was born in Oldham General Hospital. This might not seem a terribly important event except, of course, for the parents and family who were welcoming a new baby into the world. This birth was, in fact, the start of a new era in science and medicine because that baby was Louise Joy Brown. Louise was the first ever baby to be born using technology called *in vitro* fertilisation (IVF).

1978 was an interesting year for other reasons, such as the introduction of the first email system and the first cellular mobile phone (which was the size and weight of a house brick). This communication technology has become pretty dominant in the 21st Century and has thankfully reduced in size and weight! It has also become important in the effective delivery of IVF. It was also the year that 'Space Invaders' hit the Earth and took over, Olivia Newton John and John Travolta were strutting their stuff in 'Grease' and the Bee Gees were 'Stayin' Alive'. On reflection, 1978 was a good year for me; I was studying in Cambridge and on a path which would lead me to being involved in the early days of IVF. I was destined to be involved in IVF for my whole career, along with my work in stem cell technology and regenerative medicine and being an academic in several Universities.

Everything seemed a little more straightforward in 1978 than our complex, information laden lives in 2021, but it is often too easy to look back on the 'good old days' with rose coloured glasses. I know that it is important to live in the moment, not in the past. Despite this, we all naturally look back at what used to be, and this is perhaps part of what it is to be human and therefore very important. It is also how Historians make their daily bread!

CONTROVERSY

The birth of Louise Brown following IVF resulted in a lot of controversy from many different people and organisations. Some people said it was just a coincidence and that Lesley Brown became pregnant naturally! Others threw their arms up in horror at the thought of 'test-tube babies', which was a terrible term invented by the newspapers. This is even more relevant when the importance of newspapers in 1978 is considered. Newspapers were very much more influential than they are today and what and how they wrote about any subject had a considerable impact on everyone. It is important to get one thing very clear from the start: The term 'test-tube baby' can and should be dismissed as irrelevant. IVF involves neither babies (these come much later in human development) nor test-tubes, so this term will not arise again in this book.

Controversy about IVF came from many directions, including from religious leaders, scientists, physicians, politicians and of course, some of the media harshly criticised the technology. Some surgeons (you know who you are!) claimed that IVF was nonsense, and that tubal surgery (re-opening of the Fallopian tubes by a surgical procedure) was the answer. It was not; tubal surgery has never worked. Vasectomy reversal is equally ineffective. Nevertheless, there were many people who had praise and admiration for the three pioneers who made this unusual birth possible. These three people were, of course, Bob Edwards, Patrick Steptoe and Jean Purdy. Jean Purdy was a nurse by training and became the second clinical embryologist (research assistant to Bob Edwards) in the world after Bob Edwards. Jean had fantastic attention to detail in her work and was critical in the development of the laboratory technology which enabled IVF to take place both for Louise Brown and in the early days of Bourn Hall Clinic. She worked with Edwards and Steptoe in both Oldham Hospital and Bourn Hall Clinic before her untimely death, resulting from malignant melanoma, in 1985. The ongoing legacy of Edwards, Steptoe and Purdy to the world is IVF and all of the related technologies. This admirable and essential teamwork should be admired and respected by everyone. It has to be said, however, that Jean Purdy has not been recognised for her important role in developing IVF until recently. She was on many of the early research papers as an author but interestingly was not an author on the 1978 paper in the medical journal, The Lancet, which described the first IVF birth. It is easy to speculate about why this happened, but it is clearly another example of women in science not receiving the recognition they truly deserve. This is something which has to change. If someone makes a big contribution to anything, then they should get recognition; their sex and status should be irrelevant.

The basic laboratory research at Cambridge University, which led to the birth of Louise Brown began in the 1960's and the clinical collaboration between Edwards, Purdy and Steptoe began in 1968. Edwards and Steptoe actually met at a conference where Patrick Steptoe was talking about his new invention called laparoscopy. Edwards realised that this was the perfect technology to use to collect human eggs, and one of the most famous partnerships in science was formed. It took 10 years of research and collaboration to achieve the first IVF birth and from that time, the technology has grown into an industry projected to be worth $37.7 billion by 2027!

The birth of Louise Brown was a moment in history where we can look back and see that this was something very special, perhaps unique, in medical science. It is on par with medical developments, such as vaccination, blood transfusion, antibiotics and organ transplantation.

OTHER OPTIONS FOR FERTILITY PATIENTS?

Prior to the birth of Louise Brown, infertility was something which had to be accepted, with patients often adopting a 'stiff upper lip' and a 'get on with it' philosophy. In previous generations, there were many people who found that they were unable to conceive, and the only real option for these people to have a family was adoption. It is estimated that at present, there are around 153 million orphans around the world. It is very unfortunate and a human tragedy, that because of laws, religion, wars and politics, very few of these orphans will ever find adoptive parents, love and happiness. This is a tragedy on a human scale, and we should all be aware that these children need parents and homes and that we are failing them by making adoption so complex and sometimes impossible. Some fertility patients may choose to adopt if treatment fails, and this is a possible route to happiness not only for the IVF patients but most importantly, for the adopted child. If adoption was easier and more commonplace, I believe that the world would be a better place.

THE FIRST FERTILITY TREATMENTS

In the very early days of IVF at Bourn Hall Clinic, the patients (both male and female) would be inpatients for up to 3 weeks. This often resulted in quite bored patients, especially in bad weather! In the summer, the grounds of Bourn Hall

Clinic were beautiful and made a summer treatment cycle much more pleasant. Afternoon tea in the grounds of the clinic in the summer was particularly popular. The male patient would be in the clinic during the day but slept elsewhere usually in the village or in nearby Cambridge. This is in contrast to the situation today where all IVF patients are exclusively treated as outpatients. The reason for the need to use an inpatient approach at Bourn Hall Clinic was because the early technology required daily blood tests, daily urine collections (to exclude the possibility of natural ovulation), daily scans and daily injections. If the urine showed that a patient was about to ovulate naturally, then she would be taken to theatre for egg collection to avoid losing the eggs. This often resulted in the need to get together a full medical and scientific team to carry out egg collections on a 24-hour basis! Laparoscopic egg collections in the middle of the night were a regular event in the early days of IVF. Current fertility staff moaning about high workloads may like to reflect on this!

The First Technology

The early IVF technology was based on a simple and yet ingenious approach. Put very simply, the female patient receives medication to make her ovaries produce more than one egg (the scientific name for an egg is an oocyte but in IVF clinics around the world, the term egg is used). These eggs were initially collected using a surgical technique called laparoscopy. This was the start of a large range of surgical treatments used widely today which are generally known as 'key-hole' surgery. The process of laparoscopy was invented by Patrick Steptoe and key-hole surgery is a second legacy that he gave to us which is often forgotten. Today laparoscopy is used for a wide range of surgical procedures from removal of the appendix to gall bladder removal and the basic principle is that developed by Patrick Steptoe. Laparoscopy requires a full surgical team, including an anaesthetist, because the patient has a general anaesthetic and is placed onto a ventilator during the procedure.

Getting back to IVF, the male patient provides semen, by masturbation when it is needed, and the semen is prepared for fertilisation by 'washing' it with culture media to concentrate the sperm it contains and to remove some of the unwanted components of semen. The eggs and sperm are then mixed together and placed in an incubator set at body temperature (37°C) overnight. The next morning, the Clinical Embryologist looks at the eggs to see if they have fertilised. A fertilised egg shows two small circular structures called pronuclei. These are the male and female DNA which will combine to make the new individual. When these pronuclei join together, a new human individual is formed with their own, unique DNA. The eggs which have fertilised then develop into embryos over the next few days in culture, forming the familiar 2 cell, 4 cell, 8 cell embryo over the first

2-3 days and then the morula (a compact ball of about 60-80 cells) on day 4 and a blastocyst (a hollow ball of about 120 cells) on day 5 of culture. Embryos can be returned to the mother (replaced or transferrred) at any stage of development from 2 cell to blastocyst. The first ever IVF treatment used an 8 cell embryo and today the there is a trend towards using blastocysts (so called day 5 transfers/replacements) in most clinics in an attempt to select the 'best' embryo to replace. In general terms, this is a good philosophy because the embryo which develops best in the laboratory may well be the embryo which has the best potential to form a baby. Please note the use of 'may' in the previous sentence because the fact is, even today, that the visual appearance of an embryo has not been shown to have a direct correlation to a positive outcome. Many patients receive embryos which 'look perfect' but sadly, a pregnancy does not result. Many patients receive embryos which 'look bad' but become pregnant and deliver a healthy baby. This illustrates the complex, multifactorial nature of fertility treatment which we are only just starting to understand.

Fertility Treatment Today

Today, we have moved forward in some areas of IVF technology (and this will be covered in detail in Chapter 6) but there is still a long, long way to go. IVF is now an outpatient only treatment with female patients giving their injections to themselves. Sometimes partners give injections if the female patient cannot bring herself to deal with needles. This situation alone has its pros and cons. This reliance on the patient to deliver her own medication correctly and safely has always been controversial in my mind and I know that some patients dislike it.

The egg collection itself is now carried out under ultrasound guidance (not laparoscopy). This means that the patient only needs to have a light sedation for the procedure, recovers in the clinic in an hour or two and goes home the same day. If serious complications arise following egg collection, then the female patient may need to be admitted to a hospital following egg collection, but this is a very rare occurrence. The laboratory technology has changed out of all recognition since the early days, mostly for the better, but unfortunately, live birth rate has not followed suit. This conundrum of how we optimise treatment to improve live birth rate is the biggest challenge in modern IVF.

Global IVF

When Bourn Hall Clinic opened in the early 1980's it was the first and only IVF clinic in the world. Patients would come from around the globe to Bourn which is a tiny village in the Cambridgeshire countryside with the biggest attraction (apart from Bourn Hall) being the Golden Lion pub opposite the drive to Bourn Hall. The female patient used to be admitted to Bourn Hall Clinic as an inpatient and the male patient had to do his best to find accommodation in the village, possibly at the Golden Lion, in the surrounding villages or even in Cambridge. The laboratory and operating theatre were portacabins on the front lawn of the Tudor manor house which was Bourn Hall. The original manor house itself was initially used as offices, kitchen, dining room, lounge area, consulting rooms and latterly as accommodation for female patients. By the late 1980's, a considerable and expensive extension was added to Bourn Hall, using bricks and finishes to match the original Tudor building. This meant that the portacabins could finally go and we had state of the art operating theatres, laboratory and wards for fertility patients. At the same time as this massive expansion of Bourn Hall Clinic, the number of IVF clinics in the UK and in the rest of the world was growing rapidly. This meant that fewer and fewer patients needed to make the journey to the UK for treatment and even those people already in the UK found that there were very often IVF clinics near to their home when needed. The time when Bourn Hall Clinic was the only option for fertility treatment was rapidly and permanently declining.

Money!

When Edwards, Steptoe and Purdy first developed IVF, there were many people who said that they should patent their technology. This was because it was clear that IVF represented a global future industry and that the value of that industry would be enormous. This was not difficult to see even by those who were the most sceptical about the new technology. Edwards, Steptoe and Purdy were true scientists in that they did not really care about patents and money. What they cared about was bringing their safe and effective technology to patients in need and bringing hope to fertility patients. It was, therefore, no surprise that they published the details about the first IVF baby in the medical journal The Lancet (sadly without Jean Purdy as an author), and they even offered to train people in the technology at Bourn Hall Clinic for no fee! I can remember many people coming to Bourn Hall Clinic in the early days, from all around the world, to see exactly what we did and to get 'hands on' experience of the whole process of IVF. In those days, we worked on a 'see one, do one, teach one' basis. My own training at Bourn Hall Clinic involved watching experienced people carry out procedures, then doing those procedures while being supervised and finally doing everything unsupervised. The emphasis was very much on practical skill and dexterity. Anyone being trained who could not cope with this pace and style was inevitably left behind and often left the clinic. Bob Edwards also kept a very discreet eye on the results created by each Clinical Embryologist and would often offer 're-training' to any Clinical Embryologist who was not meeting his high standards. Once the free knowledge had been accumulated, visitors to Bourn Hall Clinic then took it back home and many of these people set up their own profit-making IVF clinics. This was based on what they had learnt free of charge from a visit to Bourn Hall Clinic. On reflection, it might have been better for everyone involved if this training in the early days had carried some sort of a fee but what is done is done. In later years, Bourn Hall Clinic provided training courses for a fee which were very well attended and generated a welcome small income for Bourn Hall Clinic utilising their skill and experience.

It is estimated that the global IVF industry in 2026 will be worth $27 billion. There are approximately 4000-4500 IVF clinics worldwide. The cost to patients is high in most countries largely because of the technology and skilled staff needed to provide treatment. In addition, the high cost of medications needed to carry out an IVF treatment can easily double the overall cost of treatment. These medication costs are also passed on to the fertility patient. It would be nice if the big pharma producing fertility drugs would reduce their profit to help fertility patients, but this is probably too much to ask! Japan and India currently have the largest numbers of IVF clinics with an estimated 1,100 between them. IVF is now truly a global industry and fertility clinics are commonplace in most countries. Despite this, the quality and effectiveness of the service provided varies considerably.

'Breakthroughs'

IVF has become a global phenomenon which, when it was first carried out, was headline news throughout the world. This is comparable to things such as the first heart transplant by Christian Barnard which was headline news at the time but is now commonplace. IVF is now routine and most certainly does not reach the news unless a new 'breakthrough' is announced (which is usually hype rather than fact). These 'breakthroughs' in IVF are sadly usually either unproven or simply a slight variation on what went before with no real benefit to the patient. Journalists take note! The outcome of these 'breakthroughs' is usually either small or non-existent and everyone just bumbles along as they have done since 1978. IVF needs a big kick to bring it into the 21st century and to provide a better service to all fertility patients. This will come when new leaders emerge who have the insight, bravery and imagination of Edwards, Steptoe and Purdy to change what in my opinion, has become stagnated technology. Such change will bring new, vibrant and most importantly, more successful technology. This will be the true Fertility Promise.

Nobel Prize

In 2010, Bob Edwards was awarded the Nobel Prize for his work in the development of IVF. Sadly, Patrick Steptoe and Jean Purdy had passed away and could not receive the Nobel Prize posthumously. It is also highly like that Jean

Purdy may not have qualified for the Nobel Prize because she was not an author on the first Lancet paper describing IVF. We will sadly never know. Bob Edwards was equally sadly in the grip of senile dementia when the Nobel Prize was awarded to him and so his wife Ruth travelled to Stockholm to receive the award on his behalf. It is sad that the IVF pioneers did not know that their innovative work had been recognised at the highest level. Nevertheless, it gave great reassurance to many fertility patients and immediate colleagues of Patrick, Bob and Jean, like myself that their work was unique and that it has been an enormous benefit to mankind.

Still Not A Cure

It is important to understand that IVF is not a cure for infertility. It is a process by which infertility can be 'by-passed' to achieve a pregnancy; the underlying cause of infertility does not change. It is also important to understand that 'new' technology such as egg freezing when young does not guarantee a pregnancy later in life, this is discussed in detail in Chapter 10. Fertility patients retain their initial causes of infertility. If they are successful, with live birth, and then want further children in the future, then IVF is still their only option. The only exception to this is that some females suffering from endometriosis find that pregnancy helps to reduce or even remove the endometriosis. Some of these patients may become naturally fertile as a result but certainly not all of them.

In my opinion, this makes infertility a *symptom* and not a disease. This is a controversial view, especially in N. America where infertility has to be considered a disease to be eligible for support by medical insurers. I propose that it is the various diseases (*e.g.*, tubal damage, endometriosis, male infertility, *etc.*) which cause the *symptom* of infertility. This is really an academic argument from the point of view of the fertility patient, but it is an interesting debate and one which no doubt will continue for many years to come.

Population Growth

At the time of writing, there had been at least 8 million babies born worldwide using IVF since 1978, and there are at least an additional 400,000 embryos (possibly many more) which have been frozen for possible later use. These figures are, of course, constantly increasing and contribute to the inevitable total global population in the future of 10 billion plus. It is the responsibility of everyone to ensure that the birth rate does not exceed the death rate on a global scale if we are to maintain equilibrium on planet Earth. There were, for example, over 640,000 births in the UK in 2019, with approximately 1.65 children per woman in the UK. There were 604,000 deaths in the UK in 2019, making the birth rate higher than the death rate. This means that in the UK alone, there is a steady growth in the population, not an equilibrium, and in other countries, there are similar or higher birth *versus* death data. It is also important to note that life expectancy continues to increase with many people expecting to live to 80-100 years old and some living beyond 100 years thanks to advances in modern medicine. It is the responsibility of everyone to be aware of the population dynamics of the human race on planet Earth if future generations are to have the space, food and resources needed to live. This global population problem is not directly attributable to IVF technology, but it undoubtedly contributes to the overall birth rate. The current practice of single embryo transfer in the UK and some other countries aims to not only reduce the multiple pregnancy rate which has a massive impact on the health service but also to try to keep the birth to death ratio in equilibrium. The future of the human race depends on the proper management of birth and death and may be the ultimate challenge we face in the future.

ADOPTION

The other side of this fertility coin is that there are approximately 153 million orphans in the world who need adoption with another 5,700 added to this total on a *daily basis*. This represents human suffering on a gigantic scale which most of us choose to ignore. These orphans are desperate for adoption into a loving and caring family. If fertility patients around the globe considered the possibility of adoption, then this would take hundreds of thousands of desperate orphans out of a life of misery into a life of happiness and love. This is of course easier said than done. There are many barriers to international adoption but with co-operation, understanding and determination some of these orphans could find a happy home for the rest of their lives and reduce the demand for fertility services.

PIONEERING TIMES

The early days of IVF in Bourn Hall Clinic were pioneering times because the treatment was still very new and there was still much to learn about male and female infertility and how to best handle human embryos in the laboratory. The lessons learnt from the work in Cambridge and Oldham resulting in the birth of Louise Brown would change out of recognition in the coming years. The overall live birth rate in those early days was around 30% when considering all age groups and all diagnoses. This overall live birth rate has not changed since these early days despite the efforts to improve it and despite the fact that some clinics make unsupported claims of high live birth rates by manipulating statistics. The laboratory technology at Bourn Hall Clinic was entirely manual and all of the reagents and culture media were prepared at Bourn Hall Clinic by embryologists using starting materials purchased largely from scientific suppliers and even the local chemist shop. This meant that the possibility of errors and contamination was relatively high when compared to modern media and reagents which are produced by specialised companies to clinical grade.

BLACK MONDAY

One of the reagents commonly used in IVF from the very start to today is liquid paraffin. This is layered over the culture media containing the embryos to prevent evaporation. In the early days at Bourn Hall Clinic, this liquid paraffin was simply purchased in 5 litre bottles from a pharmacy in Cambridge. Staff, including myself, quite often picked up a bottle of paraffin when visiting Cambridge to use at Bourn Hall Clinic. When the liquid paraffin arrived at Bourn Hall Clinic it was equilibrated with culture media in a bottle and 5% carbon dioxide in air was passed through it to ensure full equilibration and stability of the acidity/alkalinity known as pH. This process went very well and seemed to be safe and effective. This was until one Monday morning when we came to the laboratory and found that all of the embryos were dead. At Bourn Hall Clinic, this day became known as 'Black Monday'. Everyone was totally shocked and of course the patients involved had to be offered full refunds, a free treatment cycle and our sincere apologies. The investigation which followed showed that the cause of the toxicity on Black Monday was a batch of 'toxic' liquid paraffin. This event caused a change in the mind-set of everyone carrying out IVF and today reagents such as liquid paraffin are manufactured to the highest clinical grade specifications. There is always some level of risk in any clinical procedure, but this hard learnt lesson shows that even the most brilliant minds can and do make mistakes.

INPATIENTS AND REGULATION

The fertility treatment at Bourn Hall Clinic was at the beginning on an inpatient basis for the female patient who stayed at Bourn Hall Clinic for up to 3 weeks during treatment. She had daily ultrasound scans, bloodwork and tests of urine during this time. The male patient lived either locally in the village of Bourn or in nearby Cambridge. He could join his partner in the clinic during the day. This was a great boost for the pub in the tiny village of Bourn! At this time, it was already possible to freeze human embryos and frozen donor sperm was available if the male had insufficient sperm for *in vitro* fertilisation. It is easy to look back with rose tinted glasses but these early days of IVF in my opinion were the best in terms of the overall level of patient care and the levels of true innovation.

In the mid-to-late 1980's, the regulation of IVF began to develop in the UK following the report of the Warnock Commission which reported on how IVF should be regulated. Regulation in the UK began with the Interim Licensing Authority which was not based on legislation and was a voluntary process. This then blossomed into the Human Fertilisation and Embryology Authority (HFEA) which regulates IVF based on Human Fertilisation and Embryology Act 1990 (subsequently revised in 2008). There are now regulatory organisations in most Countries which ensure the safety of patients and the efficacy of treatment. This high level of regulation is critical in assisted reproduction to ensure that patients are protected and that the service provided to patients is of the highest possible quality.

MORE RECENTLY

The process of IVF is now provided by all clinics on a totally outpatient basis. Female patients visit the clinic for their monitoring scans, and they administer their own medication by injection, tablet and pessary (medication placed into the vagina). The egg collection is carried out under light sedation and the patient goes home later that day. She then returns for the embryo replacement (sometimes called a transfer) and carries out a home pregnancy test when the time comes to see if the treatment worked. This places a considerable additional burden on the female patients which everyone who provides IVF would do well to carefully think about. Many female patients feel stressed during their stimulation cycle often because of the requirement for self-medication. The amount of pressure placed on the female patient in modern IVF is considerable and is under-estimated by most fertility clinics. The role of the male is less in that he is only needed to produce a semen sample on the day of egg collection. This of course is a pretty critical role from a biological viewpoint! It is even possible to freeze semen before the treatment cycle and I have been involved in many IVF treatments where the male partner was overseas at the time of the treatment. This leaves the female patient even more vulnerable and in my opinion is a very bad idea. If a male cannot take time off for his own fertility treatment, then in my mind this raises serious questions about his commitment to the treatment. The male patient is of course also a critical source of support for the female patient but often neither can cope very well with the pressures put upon them. This detachment of the male and female patient in the process and the demands put onto the female patient in particular does nothing for the overall success of the treatment. Everyone agrees that a stressed patient means a patient who is less likely to succeed although it is not properly understood as to why this may be. The delivery of modern IVF means that stress levels are potentially high for all patients. In addition, there are patients who attend fertility clinics with 'infertility' who are immediately placed on an IVF treatment cycle. No consideration is taken of the general and mental health of the patients or whether or not simple interventions such as weight loss or life-style changes may significantly increase their chances of achieving a natural pregnancy. Even those patients with idiopathic (unknown cause) infertility find themselves going directly to IVF when a more simple and considerably cheaper artificial insemination procedure might be all that they need. The drive to go for a high profit IVF cycle is irresistible to the clinics and this is another area for some serious soul searching by those running IVF clinics. It is a sad fact that many fertility patients undergo expensive and invasive treatment and diagnostic procedures which they do not need in the quest to start a family and that this is a direct result of poor advice from IVF clinics. IVF clinics must change their way of thinking and not simple place everyone who walks through their door directly onto an IVF treatment cycle.

INNOVATION

Moving forward in embryology the next big innovation in IVF was Intracytoplasmic Sperm Injection (ICSI). This was originally developed to use for male patients who did not produce enough sperm for IVF and for those patients who had enough sperm for IVF but still suffered failed fertilisation in a previous IVF treatment. In this context ICSI was a great innovation. The drawbacks were that it involves considerable manipulation of human gametes, it requires additional training for clinical embryologists to become competent in the technique and the equipment required for the microinjection is expensive. As a result, when ICSI was offered it involved a significant extra cost to patients, commonly an extra cost of £1000 and sometimes even more. *Today, ICSI is the most overused technique in modern IVF*. Many clinics boast that they use ICSI in almost all patients and patients see this as a good thing because of the way in which it is sold to them as a 'guarantee' of fertilisation. The means that patients who have no clinical need for ICSI still undergo ICSI at considerable additional cost. The fertilisation 'guarantee' is also false marketing as it is well known that failed fertilisation is still possible despite using ICSI. The use of medical technology which is not clinically indicated is not allowed in all other areas of clinical practice so why does this happen in IVF? This is like telling someone with an ingrowing toe-nail that they need a leg amputation! This behaviour of fertility clinics must stop.

PROFIT AND 'ADD-ONS'

The problems in IVF sadly revolve around the development of IVF as a profit-making procedure. There is nothing inherently wrong with this as there are many other private medical clinics and hospitals offering other treatments for profit. Nevertheless, in IVF there are now thousands of private IVF clinics worldwide and some of these are 'mega' clinics who treat thousands of patients *per annum* and generate a massive income. This income is enhanced considerably in all clinics by optimising the use of ICSI (even when it is not clinically indicated) and the random and pointless use of 'add-ons' which is discussed later in this book.

This is unethical and an exploitation of vulnerable fertility patients who trust the advice they get from clinics.

Following on from the over-use of ICSI there are currently many more so called 'add-ons' which are offered to patients to allegedly increase their overall chances of a live birth. There are too many of these from 'embryo glue' to 'endometrial scratching' but the problem is that none of these 'add-ons' have been proven to be effective so once again we have IVF clinics exploiting the hopes and fears of fertility patients. Perhaps the most ridiculous and expensive of these 'add-ons' is technology which involves creating a time-lapse video of embryonic development and then claiming that this video will enable the clinical embryologist to select the 'best' embryo to replace into the mother. The equipment needed to create such a video is extremely expensive and the additional fee to the patients is high. The overall benefit of this technology to live birth rate is zero. This use of 'add-ons' in IVF is a scandal ready to break and when it does there may be many lawsuits from angry patients who have paid money for pointless procedures and technology for many years.

STAGNATION

In my opinion, IVF today has stagnated with no real increase in live birth rate but ever-increasing profits for private clinics. Part of the reason for this may be that some private clinics are owned by large corporations and others are run independently by profit focussed businessmen with little thought or empathy for fertility patients. Patient feedback often reflects this lack of compassion by some private clinics and some patients are beginning to question the ever-increasing cost of treatment especially in relation to the poor improvement in live-birth rate. The only way forward from now on is a complete change in mind-set of those people running IVF clinics to return to ethical, honest practice where nothing is offered unless it has a proven benefit to the patient. This will mean that the profit generated by IVF clinics will decrease and there is not surprisingly strong resistance to such changes. Despite this, all healthcare professionals have a duty of care to their patients which means they must only do things which will benefit the patient. At present in IVF the only people benefitting are the clinics. This is not the legacy which Edwards, Steptoe and Purdy left us, and it is time that someone spoke out to protect their legacy and to protect fertility patients. Patient care is paramount in clinical practice but unfortunately not always in IVF.

THE FUTURE

Despite these dire current problems in IVF, I think that there is an interesting and promising future for IVF. The first thing which needs to happen is a complete revision and update of the technology used in the embryology laboratory to move away from manual, error prone, procedures to true automation. This is not a time-lapse video of a developing embryo regardless of what enthusiastic manufacturers might tell you. This is technology which can bring together egg and sperm, allow fertilisation, properly monitor this process by assessing the quality and components in the culture media and perhaps using artificial intelligence to decide which are the embryos most likely to form a pregnancy. Such an approach will remove human error and human variation which will result in a more reproducible, and hopefully more successful, treatment. In addition, we need much more understanding of the process of implantation and how to optimise it to optimise live birth rate. This could be achieved either by medication or by new technology. Developing new technology for the processing, handling and understanding of sperm is needed. This technology has not really changed since 1978 and it is a glaring problem to anyone with even a basic understanding of IVF. This revolution in sperm technology will not just mean some sort of automated ICSI. It will mean a new level of understanding on both the physiology and pathology of sperm and a considerable improvement in the technology used to prepare sperm for IVF. The selection of 'good' sperm and the rejection of 'bad' sperm would be a good basic starting point. This will first need more basic research to redefine what we mean by 'good and bad' sperm based on scientific measurements and not simply on appearance. Considerably more research is needed in male infertility to allow future progress in the overall treatment of fertility.

These and many other developments may bring IVF into the 21st century instead of wallowing in the 20th century with the only focus being corporate profit. It is also likely that even with perfect embryology, andrology and clinical practice that the success rate of IVF may still not increase. This could be because the success rate we see (about 30%) is that which is defined by nature and no human intervention, no matter how advanced, can change it. If this proves to be true, then patients will have to accept that a 70% failure rate of IVF is to be expected because even the most brilliant minds cannot change things which are inevitable and the very basis of nature.

I believe that the practice of IVF today is at an all-time low because of the factors I have described above. Those providing IVF need to think carefully about the service they are offering and whether or not this service is always in the best interests of their patients. Research scientists need to receive the funding and facilities needed to develop new, safe and effective technology for IVF. Investment is needed by institutions and companies to support research. This future development will need collaboration between Universities and private clinics and Government support. Edwards, Steptoe and Purdy left us an amazing legacy; my plea is that we do not ruin this legacy by greed, unethical practice and a complete blindness to the future.

KEY POINTS OF CHAPTER 1

- The development of IVF brought controversy from many sides.
- There are many interventions for infertility and IVF is just another treatment.
- The corporate IVF industry has become a global giant, and this is not in the best interests of fertility patients.
- Contemporary IVF treatment has stagnated, and many changes are needed to get the excitement and innovation in IVF started once more.
- There is hope for IVF but there is a lot to do.
- IVF was once an inpatient procedure with no regulation; things have changed!

CHAPTER 2

The Female Patient

Peter Hollands

(The Diseases, Hopes, Wishes and Prayers for Female Patients)

> *The question isn't who is going to let me; it's who is going to stop me.*
> ***Ayn Rand***

Summary: This chapter reviews the fertility problems which can cause infertility in the female. There are many complex structural and physiological problems which can result in infertility. A better understanding of the diseases which cause infertility is important for any patient undergoing fertility treatment.

INTRODUCTION

The female fertility patient has, in my opinion, by far the toughest role to play in IVF when compared to what is required of the male. There are many reasons for this which I will cover below, but even in natural conception, the female gets the short straw because she has to carry the baby, give birth, breast feed the baby if this is the chosen option and very often be the main carer for the baby in the early years. Conception and birth can, of course, result in career disruption and many negative issues for the female. These events of human reproduction bring not only physical demands on the female but also considerable psychological stress which may even manifest into post-natal depression or the lesser 'baby blues'. This physical and psychological stress is magnified when undergoing IVF and is arguably most intense for the female. This is not to say that IVF is not stressful for the male, but perhaps that it is a different type of stress. It is important to note that the underlying disease resulting in infertility can lie with either the male or the female or with both. The overall result in any scenario will be infertility for the couple. It is important to understand that infertility is not the 'fault' of either the male or the female. This is a very real source of stress for some fertility patients. These feelings of 'blame' might be thoughts which are not openly expressed, but if it is understood by everyone that there can be no blame related to fertility then this will help. Blame has no part to play in infertility treatment. You are in this together and together you stand your best chances of success. Patients who attempt to lay blame for infertility are only creating more unnecessary stress, and such a mind-set may result in things much greater than infertility.

FEMALE INFERTILITY

Blocked Tubes

There are many reasons why a female may become infertile. Perhaps the most simple and common cause of infertility is generally known as 'blocked tubes'. The tubes which are referred to are the Fallopian tubes which pick up the egg when it is released from the ovary and take it towards the uterus (womb). Fertilisation of the egg by the sperm takes place in the tubes, and the fertilised egg will then complete its' journey along the tubes and implant into the uterus (womb) and develop into a baby. As fertilisation actually takes place in the Fallopian tubes, this demonstrates that they are not simply a tube to carry the egg, but they play a critical part in the establishment of a pregnancy. Fallopian tubes have a complex and delicate structure which is not fully understood even today. Lesley Brown, the mother of the first IVF baby Louise Brown, suffered from 'blocked tubes'. This meant that Lesley Brown was the ideal patient for the first IVF. There were no sperm problems and Lesley was completely normal apart from blocked tubes. Prior to IVF, there were many surgeons who claimed that they could surgically open 'blocked tubes' and restore fertility. These claims never materialised, and many women underwent unnecessary and ineffective tubal surgery before IVF became fully established. This is another scandal in fertility but it is out of the scope of this book.

Endometriosis

Perhaps the second most common cause of infertility is a disease known as endometriosis. This disease results from the material (blood and tissue) produced by the womb during menstruation getting into the abdomen, where it stays and grows during each menstrual cycle. This endometriosis may sit on any abdominal organ, including the ovaries and it causes pain (sometimes severe pain). Endometriosis often results in infertility, especially when the endometriosis is on the tubes or the ovaries. Endometriosis can be removed surgically but it tends to re-grow over time and surgery is ineffective in restoring fertility. Endometriosis can be treated with medication, but this simply hides the symptoms and make conceiving impossible. Most physicians agree that the real cure for endometriosis is pregnancy. In fact, several women who have had IVF babies and previously suffered from endometriosis report that their endometriosis symptoms decline following the birth of the baby and many find that they are then naturally fertile. A vicious cycle seems to be broken!

Polycystic Ovary Syndrome (PCOS)

Another form of female infertility, which has been found to respond very well to IVF, is called polycystic ovary syndrome (PCOS). In this disease, the patient develops lots of very small follicles in the ovary during each menstrual cycle. Not all of these follicles will contain an egg. This means that the physical space in the ovary for a 'normal' follicle containing an egg to develop is greatly reduced which then leads to infertility. Patients suffering from PCOS are quite commonly overweight and have increased body hair. There is no known treatment for PCOS, so the best chance of a pregnancy for these patients comes from IVF.

Thyroid

The thyroid gland is in the front of the neck and it produces many hormones which regulate the metabolism of the body. Classically an over-active thyroid results in a patient who is often thin and seems to have never ending energy. An under-active thyroid results in a patient who is often very lethargic and maybe over-weight.

An under-active or over-active, thyroid gland can prevent ovulation which in turn results in infertility. There are treatments available to correct thyroid problems and often, these are sufficient to restore fertility. It is therefore important that all female fertility patients have a blood test to screen for thyroid problems *before* going forward with IVF. In some cases, even with thyroid treatment, fertility does not return. These patients may then have to go on to IVF. Screening for thyroid problems before going forward to IVF can potentially save a lot of money and reduce the stress of infertility for some patients. It must be noted, however, that if a patient has thyroid problems plus another problem causing infertility (*e.g.*, blocked tubes) then thyroid treatment alone will not restore fertility.

Premature Menopause

All females eventually stop producing eggs in a process called menopause. The menopause usually occurs between 40-50 years of age and for some people the process is fairly uneventful. Some people suffer a wide range of symptoms at menopause, such as hot flushes, headaches and poor sleep patterns. In these patients, it is possible to provide Hormone Replacement Therapy (HRT) which often reduces or removes the symptoms of menopause.

There is a group of women who suffer what is known as premature menopause and these women undergo the same physical changes but are considerably younger, sometimes in their twenties and thirties. These young women who undergo premature menopause become infertile and the only possible intervention for them is IVF. This IVF treatment would involve hormone replacement therapy to 're-start' their ovaries and then ovarian stimulation medication to promote egg production. This approach sometimes works but not always. Those patients for whom this does not work would have to consider using donor eggs to achieve a pregnancy.

Surgical Damage and Fibroids

Gynaecological and pelvic surgery is quite common for a range of problems and surgery can often lead to scar tissue formation. This scar tissue may very easily damage or block the Fallopian tubes which results in infertility. Some women may undergo surgery on the cervix (the neck of the womb) which once again can cause scar damage or shortening of the cervix which once again may result in infertility. A damaged cervix can also lead to problems when the woman is pregnant and can even result in miscarriage in some women. Women who become pregnant with known cervical damage are closely monitored during pregnancy. The cervix may also produce mucous, which is toxic to sperm and is, therefore, a type of infertility. In all of these cases, IVF is a good option to achieve pregnancy and a live-birth.

Fibroids are non-malignant growths which occur in the womb and when they are present, the embryo may have little or no physical room to implant and to form a baby. Fibroids can be removed surgically, and women may then go on to have a natural conception. IVF is an option for those women who have had fibroids removed who may also have other causes of infertility as well as fibroids or their partner has associated male infertility. The development of fibroids appears to be more common in Sub-Sahara Africa but at present it is not known why women from this part of the world are more prone to fibroids.

Sterilisation

There are millions of women throughout the world who have undergone surgical sterilisation by having clips placed on the Fallopian tubes which result in blocked tubes. This process is often used as a method of family planning but some women who have been surgically sterilised later decide that they want more children. Some surgeons may offer to remove the clips in the hope that the Fallopian tubes will re-open but, in most cases, this is unsuccessful due to damage to the tubes by the clips and scarring. Patients who have had their tubes surgically blocked as a means of sterilisation are therefore very often seen in IVF clinics around the world. Such patients should fare well in IVF because they often have proven fertility. This is, of course, assuming that the female patient is ideally well below the age of 40 when IVF treatment is used. Patients aged 40 and above fare very badly in IVF treatment (1-2% success rate).

Medications

There are a few medications and medical procedures which have the unfortunate consequence of causing infertility or sub-fertility (reduced fertility). These include such medications as long-term, high dose use of ibuprofen, aspirin, anti-psychotics or fluid retention medication such as spironolactone which can reduce fertility. This does not mean that you should stop taking any prescribed medication because you think it might be causing infertility. This must be discussed with the prescribing physician and also a physician at your IVF clinic. *Please do not make any changes to your medication without specific instructions from the doctor treating you.* High dose chemotherapy and radiotherapy to treat cancer will cause ovarian failure and infertility. Many such patients opt to freeze their eggs at an IVF clinic prior to undertaking chemotherapy or radiotherapy in the hope that later on in life, when the chemotherapy is out of the body, they may be able to have children using their frozen eggs. This is by far not a guarantee of a future pregnancy following chemotherapy or radiotherapy but it provides hope for some patients.

Other Causes of Infertility

There is good evidence that illegal drug use can lead to infertility or sub-fertility in both men and women. Experience has also shown that excessive alcohol intake, smoking and obesity can severely affect fertility. The message here is simple: To optimise fertility, do not use illegal drugs, do not drink *excessive* amounts of alcohol (ideally no alcohol at all), do not smoke at all and ensure that you have a healthy diet and regular exercise to avoid obesity. These simple measures can very often result in a return to fertility with no requirement for IVF at all. These actions will also greatly improve your overall quality of life and save you a lot of money! This advice applies to all fertility patients (and indeed to my other patient cohort of people wanting stem cell treatment) regardless of whether or not IVF is planned to be used in the future.

Idiopathic Infertility

Idiopathic infertility means that the cause of the infertility is unknown, and all current testing cannot show any abnormality which may result in infertility. This does not mean that the cause is not there, it is simply unknown. This diagnosis of idiopathic appears across clinical medicine and it is a sobering reminder that we all still have a great deal to learn. The symptoms of infertility in idiopathic infertility are still very real and very distressing. The treatment for idiopathic infertility is IVF but it should be preceded by artificial insemination whenever possible. The treatment for infertility with a clear cause is also IVF and this may even be preceded by artificial insemination if the Fallopian tubes are open, and the sperm count is good. The treatments are the same regardless of the diagnosis. During the IVF treatment of idiopathic infertility more information may come to light, such as poor egg quality or sperm, which look normal but are unable to fertilise the egg. This is quite a common observation and it illustrates very well that 'normal looking' eggs and sperm are not necessarily normal. If such discoveries are made, the subsequent treatment cycles may involve treatment or technology (*e.g.*, ICSI) to get around these problems. It is estimated that 39% of all fertility patients have an idiopathic diagnosis and a great many of these may have success, in terms of producing a pregnancy and birth by use of simple artificial insemination rather than IVF. Some of the best clinics offer 3-6 artificial insemination treatment cycles before progressing onto IVF. This saves considerable time and money and reduces stress for the patients. As time and technology progresses, the diagnosis of idiopathic infertility may decrease because of advances in knowledge and in technology resulting in more clear diagnoses. This may allow more currently unknown (idiopathic) causes of infertility to be attributed to a specific cause and treated accordingly. This will reduce the number of patients who today are classed as suffering from idiopathic infertility, which is a stressful diagnosis for anyone to receive because of the sense of the unknown.

Stress!

At the start of this chapter, I mentioned that the female patient has the toughest role to play in IVF from a physical point of view. Most people would agree with this assertion. The physical challenges on the female are only too familiar to fertility patients. These include many investigations, including blood tests, ultrasound scans, the invasive surgical collection of eggs and the transfer of the developing embryo back into the womb. Despite this, it is also important to consider the emotional and psychological impact of infertility and IVF treatment which are arguably now more significant than the physical challenges. The worries begin from that start: Will I be accepted for IVF? Will I administer my injected medication correctly? If not, what will happen? Will I respond to ovarian stimulation? Will I over respond to ovarian stimulation? Will sufficient eggs be collected? Will the eggs fertilise? Will the embryos develop well? Will I get an embryo transfer? Will any embryos be frozen? Will I become pregnant? Will the pregnancy go to term? Will the baby be normal? These and many other worries and thoughts pile on the psychological pressure for all fertility patients. The best way to deal with these questions and worries is to optimise knowledge about the process of fertility treatment and to avoid social media or online 'experts' on the subject of infertility.

Then there is the dreaded '2 week wait' from embryo transfer to pregnancy test which is arguably the most stressful part of any IVF treatment cycle for both the male and the female. At the end of the 2 week wait, the patient carries out a pregnancy test so see if the fertility treatment has worked. Perhaps the biggest worry of all is what will I do if the pregnancy test is negative? The options are to try again with considerable associated cost, give up and accept that you will never have children or consider alternatives such as adoption. These are important life-changing decisions which must never be made in isolation. Fertility patients should talk to clinic staff, including the counsellor, in the decision process.

'BACK-TO-BACK' TREATMENTS

Most fertility patients get tied up in the never-ending cycle of IVF treatment cycles, often in consecutive months. This 'back-to-back' fertility treatment should be avoided at all costs. It can cause physical and emotional stress which can be very damaging. The momentum for 'back-to-back' treatments often comes from fertility patients themselves as when they receive a negative outcome, they feel pressure not to 'waste time' and want to get on with another treatment. Most patients find that a break between treatments is very welcome from a physical and psychological point of view, some even fall pregnant naturally during the break!

I have even seen patients who had undergone many treatment cycles without any success and made the final decision to stop treatment totally and go on holiday. They then got pregnant naturally on holiday. IVF is not always the answer.

These factors all add up to considerable psychological stress for the female patient which can be shared to some extent with her partner, her family, the clinic staff and sometimes the clinic counsellor. The clinic counsellor is very much underused by most fertility patients and this person is a great resource if only as a friendly ear. Please use your clinic counsellor more. He/she is a very valuable resource to you as patient and utilising the counsellor is not a sign of weakness, it is a sign of intelligence and awareness, and the discussions you have may be very helpful.

Another point of stress arises if the female patient is in full-time employment during the IVF treatment cycle. If this is the case, the female patient will need to take time out on several occasions during the treatment for scans, blood tests and consultations. An un-supportive employer can cause another level of stress which is very unwelcome. My suggestion is that you discuss your plans with a trusted person where you are employed so that each party understands clearly what is happening and you get the support you need. Most employers will support women undergoing fertility treatment, but they can only do this if the patients tell them about their treatment and the demands it will make on their time and emotions.

It is important to note that stress releases hormones which can actually reduce fertility levels in some people. There is a hormone called prolactin which is raised in stress and can inhibit ovulation. There are, no doubt, many other factors present in a stressed person which could impact on fertility. It is therefore very important to try to minimise stress during your treatment cycle. A happy patient may equal a happy outcome!

A FINAL PRAYER

The prayer of every female fertility patient is that all of this discomfort and stress which comes with fertility treatment will lead to a normal pregnancy and the birth of a perfect baby. It sounds like a simple request but IVF is in fact a very complicated process with low success rates. It is important to understand that 70% of IVF treatment cycles result in no pregnancy. Even if a pregnancy is established, then it may not go to term in the same way as any naturally conceived pregnancy. These may seem to be unwelcome negative thoughts but to get through fertility treatment (and to retain your sanity!) you have to accept the hard truth about what you are trying to do. If IVF works (30% of the time), it brings joy and happiness to both the parents and to the clinic staff. It is the best part of the job when patients achieve a pregnancy. If IVF does not work (70% of the time), it brings sadness and sometimes despair to the patients. There is a parallel feeling of loss and inadequacy in the clinic staff who often question their decisions and judgment when a negative result occurs. Please think about these things beforehand and make yourself fully aware of what you are trying achieve and the risks involved. This will make things easier to handle if things do not go to plan.

It is also good advice to take each day as it comes when going through fertility treatment and to keep expectations realistically low. Once again this is not to encourage negativity but to encourage realism. There are so many 'hurdles' in a fertility treatment, some fall at the first, some fall at the last, but always keep in mind that only 30% of patients will clear all of the 'hurdles'. This will avoid severe disappointment and may even help you to cope better with the process.

KEY POINTS OF CHAPTER 2

- There are many diseases in the female which can result in infertility. Your clinic will assess you thoroughly and come to a diagnosis.
- Some patients suffer idiopathic infertility where a cause cannot be identified.
- Stress can have a negative impact on fertility treatment and every effort should be made to reduce stress as much as possible.
- Be optimistic during your fertility treatment but at the same time be realistic.

CHAPTER 3

The Male Patient

Peter Hollands

(The Diseases, Hopes, Wishes and Prayers for Male Patients)

Being a male is a matter of birth. Being a man is a matter of choice.
Edwin Louis Cole

Summary: This chapter considers the various causes of male infertility and the input of the male into the overall process of fertility treatment. Fertility treatment is unique in that it involves 2 patients at the same time and the role of these patients is equally important to the overall success of the treatment. The male plays a critical role in fertility treatment, and this role may be down-played by some fertility clinics to the point at which the male feels disengaged from the treatment process. This is a bad thing.

INTRODUCTION

It is clear that the male patient in fertility treatment has a critical role to play in the overall success of fertility treatment. Nevertheless, some male patients often feel 'left out' or not really part of the process because of the great focus on the female patient. This is something which most IVF clinics fully understand but few, if any, have a clear strategy to support male patients. I believe that better support for male patients would result in better overall success of fertility treatments and happier female patients.

THE MALE ROLE IN FERTILITY TREATMENT

The primary role of the male patient in fertility treatment is to provide a semen sample by masturbation on the day of egg collection. This is so that his sperm can be used to fertilise the surgically collected eggs from his partner in the laboratory. This may sound a little stark, but these are the hard facts. The male of course also has the critical role of supporting his partner through fertility treatment. This is much more subtle, and I believe that it is key to the overall well-being of both patients during treatment and possibly even the optimum outcome of the treatment process. Many men are under extreme stress during fertility treatment, especially on the day of egg collection, but many do not share these worries and concerns with anyone. Some of the very best fertility clinic staff may notice these male anxieties and offer re-assurance but this kind of support for the male patient is far from common. This male mind-set sadly is typical of the male psyche which always tends to resist support and advice even when it may be desperately needed. Despite this, a supportive and understanding male patient will enhance the experience of fertility treatment for his partner and may even, in turn enhance the outcome. The male patient should not feel 'left out', but he should feel that he is an integral part of the whole fertility treatment process in the same way as in natural conception.

THE 'MEN'S ROOM' PORNOGRAPHY AND SEMEN ASSESSMENT

The key process in establishing the fertility of a male is for an experienced Clinical Embryologist to examine a semen sample in detail in the IVF laboratory in a fertility clinic. This requires the male to produce a semen specimen by masturbation in what is usually known in most fertility clinics as the 'men's room'. This is usually a room in a quiet part of the clinic which contains washing facilities (some of the best have a shower) and a selection of pornographic magazines and videos. Some clinics will allow the partner of the man to go to the men's room with him, but this may not be possible especially on the day of egg collection where the partner is likely to be in theatre. Many clinics also have homosexual pornography available, especially those who treat many homosexual couples. I have had many male patients complain about the 'quality' of the pornography provided in the men's room and ask for more 'hardcore' material. This became such a problem in the early days at Bourn Hall Clinic that staff were sent to Amsterdam to collect more 'suitable' pornography for the men's room. It is worth remembering that this is long before the days of internet pornography. I am reliably informed that today any form of pornography can easily be obtained on a mobile phone, so this particular problem in semen production may now be solved.

In the early days of IVF, we asked male patients to produce what we called a 'split ejaculate'. The basically involved 2 collection pots sellotaped together into which the male patient had to put the first 'spurt' of the ejaculate into the first pot and the remains of the ejaculate into the second pot. The idea here was that the first 'spurt' contained the best quality sperm. As you can imagine this caused considerable stress for some male patients to the point that some were unable to ejaculate at all because of the stress of hitting the right pot. Luckily for all male patients, this fashion has long since been abolished when it was proven that a 'split ejaculate' was no better than an ejaculate collected into just one pot. Any male attending an IVF clinic today will only be asked to use one pot.

Another area where men often feel anxious or embarrassed is the point at which the embryologist shows him to the men's room. The anxiety is often heightened if the Clinical Embryologist happens to be female. The only thing that I can say about this is that the Clinical Embryologists are all highly experienced healthcare professionals who do this job day in and day out. It is part of their normal routine and is not a subject of any specific discussion or reflection. It is just a natural part of the process and there should be no embarrassment on the part of the male patient. Despite all of this, if you are still worried and would prefer a male to take you to the men's room then please tell either the nurses, embryologists, or the physicians in your clinic and it should be possible to meet your needs. If you feel any level of stress during fertility treatment, please do not bottle it up, tell the clinic staff and they will do everything they possibly can to help you.

A semen assessment carried out in a general pathology laboratory at a hospital is best avoided as the staff there will not have the experience required to make a good and reliable diagnosis. If your GP suggests this, it is best to say that you prefer to do your semen assessment at the fertility clinic. In my experience, the following sperm parameters describe the minimum quality of sperm which will result in good fertilisation *in vitro,* these are:

60 million sperm per mL (the number of sperm per mL in the ejaculate)

60% good sperm motility (the way in which the sperm swim)

60% normal sperm morphology (normal forms or appearance)

This is sometimes known as the 'rule of 60' (by me anyway!)

The sperm is diluted to approximately 100,000 per mL for the actual fertilisation of the egg using IVF. Too many sperm can 'overwhelm' the egg and more than one sperm may fertilise, which results in an abnormal embryo which cannot be used for treatment.

If the sperm parameters turn out to be less than the 'rule of 60', then IVF may still be possible but with an increased risk of failed fertilisation. If the sperm parameters are considerably less than the 'rule of 60' then interventions such as Intracytoplasmic Sperm Injection (ICSI) may be needed, which is described in detail later in this book. The key parameters of total sperm count, percentage motility and percentage normal forms give the Clinical Embryologists critical information about the likely outcome of any treatment and the type of treatment which is needed. It should be noted that scientists do not fully understand why sperm counts are different in different men and they certainly do not have the technology, at least at the time of writing, to manipulate sperm quality with either medication or other treatments. If you are offered magical procedures or medications (at great cost) which claim to manipulate sperm quality or numbers and thus increase fertility, then walk away. These offering are untested and unproven and will not improve sperm parameters. You are being deliberately misled for profit.

Hot Pants!

There is a reasonably clear relationship between an increased temperature of the scrotum and a related decline in sperm quality. This has led to some people recommending that men trying to conceive should not take hot baths and may even consider wearing loose boxer-shorts as underwear. The science behind these ideas is inconclusive but what is known is that nature has designed the male to carry the testes outside the main body. The main result of this is that the testes are kept at a lower temperature than the core body temperature. This of course does not allow for clothes, underwear and hot baths which most men may not want to give up. The best advice here is to be sensible: No hot baths, no tight underwear and no saunas but clothes are probably a good idea.

Testicular Damage

Any form of damage to the testicles will seriously affect the quality of the sperm produced by a man. This damage can come in many forms including infection, cancer, testicular surgery, congenital (inherited) disease, un-descended testicles and trauma to the testicles (*e.g.* injuries received during contact sports). There is some evidence that male cyclists are more prone to testicular problems, but this is mainly professional cyclists so a quick trip to the shops on a bike is no doubt perfectly safe. Most of these testicular problems are fairly self-explanatory apart from un-descended testicles. In normal development, the testicles form inside the abdomen of the fetus and in normal development they then 'descend' into the scrotum. In patients suffering from un-descended testicles, the testicles are retained inside the abdominal cavity and as a result the testicles exist at the normal core body temperature. This can result in damage to the testicles which may be so bad that no sperm are produced at all.

Vasectomy

A very common cause of male infertility is vasectomy. This may sound ridiculous as the point of a vasectomy is to make a man sterile. Vasectomy is a relatively simple surgical procedure under a local anaesthetic and it is usually undertaken as a method of birth control when a man has completed his family and does not want any further children. In a perfect world, this is a completely acceptable process. Unfortunately, the world is not a perfect place and many things may happen which results in a man who has had a vasectomy wanting further children. He may find another partner and want another family or his present children may die (sorry to be so blunt) and he wants further children with his existing partner. In these situations, the only options are either micro-surgery to reconnect the tubes which were cut during vasectomy or IVF. The micro-surgery to re-connect the tubes cut during vasectomy has been shown to be very unsuccessful and very few, if any, surgeons offer this option. If the male patient who has had a vasectomy goes for IVF then the sperm will have to be collected surgically by surgically aspirating the sperm directly from the testes. This will sound like horrendous torture to most men but in fact it is a relatively pain free procedure, carried out at the clinic under light sedation, and it is successful for most patients who have previously had a vasectomy. The resultant surgically collected sperm are used to fertilise the eggs of the female partner and it is highly likely that ICSI will need to be used as the fertilisation method. This is because surgical sperm collection produces fewer sperm than the numbers found in a normal ejaculate, making routine IVF impossible. The positive side of this kind of treatment is that in most cases neither the male nor female patient have fertility issues as they have almost always had children naturally prior to the IVF treatment. This means that the overall success rate in such patients may be slightly increased assuming that all other factors such as maternal age are being taken into account.

Ejaculation and Psychosexual Disorders

There are some men who for various reasons find ejaculation difficult. This may be because of a condition known as retrograde ejaculation. Men suffering from this condition do not ejaculate semen normally, but they ejaculate semen back into their own bladder. This is often because of structural problems with the tubes which carry semen from the testes to the outside world. It is often possible to treat this condition by collecting the urine which is produced after retrograde ejaculation as this urine often contains many viable sperm which can be used for IVF usually using ICSI. If this process fails, then such men will almost certainly be able to undergo surgical sperm collection with a good outcome, once again by using ICSI.

There are also some psychosexual disorders which can result in difficulty to ejaculate or difficulty in attaining an erection sufficient for masturbation. Such problems are really beyond the scope of an IVF clinic and are best handled by healthcare professionals specifically trained to help in those circumstances. There are some medications (*e.g.* Viagra) which can be easily obtained by the patient but it is better to take such medications under the guidance of a healthcare professional who will also be able to assess other underlying problems which may be associated with the difficulty in erection and/or ejaculation.

Hormonal and Genetic Disorders

The ability of a man to produce sperm capable of fertilising an egg depends on the correct balance of male hormones in the man. The most important of these hormones is testosterone. If testosterone levels are low, then sperm production will be low or non-existent and the testicles themselves are often found to be much smaller than those in a fertile man. There have been attempts to supplement testosterone in such patients, but the outcome is generally poor, presumably because the testicles have undergone some irreversible changes which increased hormone levels cannot correct. Male patients suffering from these problems may have to consider the use of donor sperm to achieve a pregnancy.

Small testicles may also be found when there is a tumour present, or the patient may be taking illegal drugs which are known to have a damaging effect on testicles and sperm production. There is also a relatively rare genetic condition called Klinefelter Syndrome where the male patient, instead of having the usual XY genetic make-up, has an XXY genetic make-up. The extra X chromosome results in poor testicular development and resultant infertility. The only hope for such patients is donor sperm. Donor sperm is a very important option in fertility treatment, but it must be used only after the patients have had chance to discuss the implications both with clinic staff and the clinic counsellor. There are many excellent donor sperm banks available to patients.

Medicines and Drugs

Medicines and drugs can affect sperm production in many ways in a similar way to how drugs and medicines can affect egg production in women. In the case of men, it is known that the prescribed medication sulfasalazine, which is an anti-inflammatory medication often used to treat Chrohn's disease and rheumatoid arthritis, can decrease the number of sperm being produced. Fortunately, the sperm production will increase once more when the medication is discontinued so no permanent damage should be done. It is worth noting however that sperm production takes about 3 months to complete in the testicles so the increase in the sperm count to normal may take some time and it will certainly not happen as soon as the medication is discontinued.

I have seen many male patients who have chosen to take anabolic steroids usually for body building purposes. The long-term use of anabolic steroids, especially out of medical supervision, often results in reduced sperm count and motility. In some patients, the sperm number and motility do not increase even after the patient stops taking anabolic steroids. There is therefore a risk of permanent damage to sperm production if anabolic steroids are used, especially without medical supervision. The basic message here is to avoid anabolic steroids at all costs if you intend to have a family in the future. Being a fertile wimp is better than being an infertile muscle man!

Chemotherapy, used in the treatment of cancer and related diseases, will almost always reduce sperm production to zero. This is because chemotherapy inhibits cell division. Any man who has to undergo chemotherapy, and wants a family in the future, should provide samples of semen for freezing before the chemotherapy begins. These samples can be frozen at any IVF clinic and they will be available at any time in the future if needed. The quality of the sperm when thawed should be sufficient to create a pregnancy by artificial insemination or by IVF with ICSI.

Herbal remedies are best avoided by men wishing to reproduce, especially root extracts of the Chinese herb *Tripterygium wilfordii* which can decrease sperm production and reduce the size of the testicles. Illegal drugs will all have significant negative effects on sperm production and must be avoided at all costs, both for fertility and general health reasons.

There are some 'over-the-counter' medications on the market which claim to be able to improve sperm quality. It is best to avoid all of these as there is no convincing scientific data which show that any of these medications have any positive effect on sperm production. They are also very expensive, and all have clever marketing. They are all a waste of money!

Life-style Issues

In the same way as the female, there are life-style issues that will affect male fertility. These are such things as excess alcohol consumption, smoking and a poor diet and exercise regime resulting in obesity. Many men who have these life-style issues and change their behaviour find that their fertility increases or returns without any further treatment. The basic message here is to be as naturally fit and healthy as you possible can without resorting to any sort of drug or medication unless it is prescribed under medical supervision. All fertility patients will be advised to reduce alcohol intake if it is needed, stop smoking and reduce obesity if needed. These changes will not only help your fertility, but they will also improve your general health.

Stress

The information on the effects of stress on male fertility is less well documented than in the female. Despite this it is clear that stress will have a considerable impact on the overall wellbeing of anyone. By reducing or minimising stress, this can not only help overall health, but also well-being and perhaps even fertility of the male. The actual IVF treatment cycle is a stressful process for anyone. To have this in mind when embarking on IVF treatment, with a strategy to minimise stress where at all possible, may be very helpful and may even improve the outcome of your treatment. Some people find yoga, meditation and sometimes acupuncture as useful methods to reduce stress but if you have any activity which you feel reduces stress then it should be utilised during fertility treatment. It will do no harm and it might even be the key to success. Some fertility clinics offer acupuncture with the idea that it will improve sperm count or make you more fertile is some way. This is not proven and you are well advised to reject such 'treatment' if it is offered in this context.

A FINAL PRAYER

The final prayer for the male fertility patient is not surprisingly the same as the female patient. The anticipated outcome is a healthy live birth and this is what everyone at a fertility clinic wishes for you. Nevertheless, as in the female, it is important to know that live birth success rates run at about 30% and that disappointment is likely to be the outcome. Please be very suspicious of fertility clinics claiming 50% success rate and sometimes even higher! These are false claims to attract fee paying patients. You are much better with a clinic who will tell you the truth, no matter how hard it might be, than a clinic who operates in a fantasy world with the main target being profit. These are hard facts to think about but being aware and realistic when undergoing fertility treatment will help you to cope better with the considerable ups and downs which you will experience. Some clinics present a far too rosy picture of fertility treatment and if this is the case then the disappointment is even tougher to handle. I must stress that I am not suggesting negativity. My suggestion is a thorough understanding of the process you will be going through combined with a well-informed and realistic approach. This will prevent severe disappointment and may even help you towards success.

KEY POINTS OF CHAPTER 3

- The male and female patients are of equal importance in fertility treatment.
- Semen analysis by an experienced clinical embryologist at a fertility clinic is very important.
- Sensible health and well-being practices will optimise sperm quality.
- Keep stress to a minimum if at all possible.

CHAPTER 4

The LGBT Patients

Peter Hollands

(How IVF Can Help Anyone to Have a Child)

It is absolutely imperative that every human being's freedom and human rights are respected, all over the world.
Jóhanna Sigurðardóttir

Summary: IVF was once only available to married heterosexual couples. This was clearly discrimination against all other patients and today, IVF technology is made available to anyone in need, including single women using donor sperm. This Chapter reviews IVF from the point of view of LGBT patients and provides some insight and advice to those patients who are either undergoing or considering this course of treatment.

INTRODUCTION

When IVF was first developed, it was reserved for heterosexual couples. Most clinics even refused to treat single women. A single woman wanting to have a child would, of course, need to obtain donor sperm for her treatment and this is described in detail in Chapter 9. Since those early days, the attitudes towards who may or may not have access to fertility treatment have changed completely. Today fertility treatment is available for anyone, including same sex female and same sex male couples. The technology needed can be more complex and it is often very much more expensive but other than that, there are no particular barriers to helping same sex couples to have a family.

SAME SEX FEMALE PATIENTS

Same sex female patients are often treated in IVF clinics. This does not mean that either partner necessarily suffers from infertility and quite often, they are both completely fertile.

There may be cases where a simple donor sperm insemination is all that is needed to achieve a pregnancy for these patients. If this is the case, then this is a relatively straightforward treatment and is certainly the first step if the partner wanting to become pregnant appears to be naturally fertile. The main decision to be made is which female partner will be inseminated and this can usually be determined by hormonal screening and ultrasound scans to assess which female partner is most likely to become pregnant. If both female partners have the same level of fertility, then either partner may receive the donor sperm with an equal chance of a good outcome. The key in this case of donor insemination is to ensure that the donor sperm is properly screened and is of the highest quality. There are many excellent donor sperm banks providing safe and high-quality donor sperm to anyone in need.

If the initial investigations indicate that neither female patient is likely to achieve a pregnancy by donor insemination (for example, if both female patients have blocked tubes or hormonal abnormalities) then it may be necessary to use IVF to achieve a pregnancy. If this is the case, then a decision has to be made about which female partner will provide the eggs for the treatment? This may be a purely medical decision based on the relative fertility of each woman, but some couples have a clear vision about who shall provide the eggs and this must always be respected. It is quite common that one partner elects to provide the eggs and the other partner elects to carry the baby but once again, this decision should be left to the patients unless there are significant medical issues to consider.

Surrogacy for Same Sex Female Patients

It is possible that neither female partner wishes to be pregnant and carry the baby, but they still want a family. If so, a surrogate mother would need to be found. This involves considerable organisation, legal implications and potentially considerable cost to the patients. It is sometimes possible for female members of the family or friends to act as a surrogate mother. If such a surrogate is proposed, then this needs careful discussions, support and counselling from the IVF clinic involved. Taking on the role of surrogate mother is a physically and emotionally straining process which should not be taken on lightly.

Female Partner Providing Eggs for Treatment

The female partner who chooses to provide the eggs for the treatment has to undergo ovarian stimulation and ultrasound egg collection as described in Chapter 6. The eggs are then fertilised using the donor sperm (often using ICSI) and the resultant embryos develop in the laboratory. Some IVF clinics have their own donor sperm banks, but if not, there are excellent donor sperm banks available who can help anyone in need. There will often be surplus embryos suitable to freeze for future treatment cycles if needed but this is not always the case. The best embryo is transferred into the female partner (or surrogate) who will carry the baby and a pregnancy test is carried out on day 14 (from the egg collection date) and if pregnant, a day 35 scan (from the egg collection date) is carried out as described in Chapter 6. The resultant pregnancy is managed by GPs, ante-natal clinics and delivery units in the same way as any other pregnancy.

SAME SEX MALE PATIENTS

Same sex male patients who wish to have a family can also be helped by the use of IVF technology. Same sex male patients will not need to obtain donor sperm (unless they both happen to suffer from male infertility which is highly unlikely) but they will definitely need the services of an egg donor and a surrogate mother. This can be very costly, but it certainly works, as people such as Elton John have shown. Some same sex male patients often choose to use a mixture of sperm from both partners to inseminate the donor eggs and this can be offered by most IVF clinics.

Egg Donation and Surrogacy

Same sex male patients have to have an egg donor and a surrogate mother in order to achieve their dream of parenthood. This increases the complexity and cost of same sex male fertility treatment, but it is not an insurmountable problem. Donor eggs cost in the region of £9,000 in the UK but this will vary from clinic to clinic. In the USA donor eggs can cost from $20,000-$40,000. The patients need to choose their egg donor very carefully. The medical history of the egg donor and her appearance and race are very important to the patients, and this must be studied and approved by both the treatment clinic and the patients. Friends and family may be egg donors, but this requires a thorough understanding of the role of the egg donor, the legal implications and any expenses payable.

In the UK, surrogate mothers cannot be paid for their service but they can be paid expenses related to the role of surrogate mother. This would include such things as loss of earnings, travel and childcare. These expenses are typically £7,000-£15,000 in the UK and $90,000 to $130,000 in the USA.

Gender Re-Assignment

Advances in surgical techniques, and in hormonal manipulation and control have enabled many people to undergo gender re-assignment in recent years. This is clearly a major life-changing process and must not be undertaken lightly. IVF clinics often have a role to play in the overall process in terms of egg or sperm collection and freezing before gender re-assignment treatment begins. The technology used for egg and sperm freezing for gender re-assignment patients is the same as that used for any other patient. The gender re-assignment patient must undergo the appropriate counselling at the IVF clinic. Once the gender re-assignment is complete, the patient may return to the fertility clinic (many years later) for treatment using previously frozen eggs and sperm.

The provision of fertility services for LGBT patients has improved considerably in the past 25 years. This progress is a great credit to the fertility clinics and the related regulatory authorities who have made the opportunity of a family for these people a reality. The cost is high, especially for same sex male couples, but apart from this drawback, no patients will be refused treatment. It is however, worth noting that some fertility clinics may not have the infrastructure or expertise needed to treat LGBT patients but if this happens, then there are many other clinics who will be able to help.

KEY POINTS OF CHAPTER 4

- Same sex female and same sex male patients can now be treated to achieve a family by most fertility clinics.
- Donor sperm, egg donors and surrogate mothers may be needed depending on the needs and preferences of the patients.
- Gender re-assignment patients often undergo gamete (egg or sperm) storage, prior to their gender re-assignment treatment, in fertility clinics.

CHAPTER 5

IVF Clinics

Peter Hollands

(The Good, The Bad and The Ugly)

Isn't it a bit unnerving that doctors call what they do "practice"?
George Carlin

Summary: This chapter assesses the IVF clinics providing fertility treatment in terms of cost and other factors which clinics use to attract fertility patients to use their services. IVF clinics around the world are mainly privately owned companies operating to make a profit. They also offer various different packages and treatments to attract fertility patients to the clinic. Some countries have public funded IVF treatment, but the availability of such treatments is restricted.

INTRODUCTION

There are thousands of IVF clinics around the world and as in any part of life some are 'better' than others. This may be a reality, or it may just be in the eye of the beholder. There are many ways in which an IVF clinic may be 'better' than others, but the patient has to navigate the marketing and hype to ensure that their chosen clinic meets their needs. Some fertility clinics have enormous marketing budgets (especially in N. America) and can therefore potentially recruit more patients for treatment. Such large clinics may also rely on 'technology' they offer or 'famous' staff to attract patients. Other smaller clinics may have to rely on website traffic or even word of mouth. The final decision on which private fertility clinic to use lies with the fertility patient. Perhaps the most telling and important information coming out of a fertility clinic is the patient feedback from patients who were treated at that specific clinic. This may be from successful patients (who may of course be naturally pleased with their treatment and turn a blind eye to any problems) but also more importantly from patients for whom treatment may have failed. If patients had a failed treatment, but still praise the treatment they received from a fertility clinic, then such a clinic might be worth a second look. It is, of course, also necessary to warn about patient testimonials as they may or may not be true. The following information may be useful in the process of selecting the 'best' fertility clinic and optimising the success of an IVF treatment cycle.

MONEY!

Most fertility patients seeking treatment around the world will find themselves speaking to a private clinic about their potential treatment. This may be the first experience of private medicine for many patients (for example patients in the UK) and the whole process can be quite daunting and confusing. Private clinics of all types have to have a minimum base income to enable them to operate. This is the same for all private IVF clinics who must cover the cost and maintenance of the building in which they operate, the cost of staff, the cost of equipment and consumables and the cost of licensing. This is basic business and is not the sole remit of private IVF clinics but applies to all private and public healthcare.

The fertility patient is, of course, very concerned and interested in how much the fertility treatment will cost. This might seem to be a simple question but the way in which fertility services are delivered makes the definitive figure difficult to tie down. This is, of course, totally unacceptable. If someone is buying a car then they might be told that the cost will be £20,000. In this cost will be everything required for the car to travel from point to point in relative comfort and safety at your will. If the same person asks the same question but this time about the cost of fertility treatment then the reply will be vague, low and totally opaque. It is almost like buying the car and then being told that you need to pay for the engine and wheels as 'add-ons'. I have driven Mercedes-Benz cars from new for over 30 years, and I can remember very clearly paying for a radio as an 'extra' in some of my early purchases. I put up with this ridiculous practice because of the badge but on reflection I was being ripped off when every other car on the market at that time came with a radio. Mercedes could have easily installed a radio and passed the hidden cost onto the customer but no, they preferred to have it as an extra. This rant may not seem relevant (and it might not be!) but a similar thing is happening all the time in fertility clinics. Patients are given a basic cost and then a massive shopping list of other costs. Even the clinics themselves often find it difficult to come up with their own total costs! This confusion and lack of transparency about the true cost of fertility treatment is a major problem which is going to be very difficult to resolve unless fertility clinics change the way in which they think and work.

In summary, it is therefore virtually impossible to give an accurate overall cost of fertility treatment but there are some basic guidelines which if exceeded should ring alarm bells and raise questions. In the UK for example the 'basic' cost of IVF is usually stated at £3-4,000. The first thing to understand here is that this overall cost will be *much higher* than this 'basic' cost. All clinics charge extra for blood tests (which can easily add up to an extra £1000 if repeated or complex blood tests are needed) and for the medication which is used in the treatment cycle which can easily cost £2000. Blood tests are almost always carried out by external specialised laboratories and can be very expensive and medication is manufactured by big pharma such as Serono and many others. This means such medications are very expensive. The IVF clinic therefore has to pay for these services and products and many IVF clinics add their own profit margin to these costs which of course comes out of the pocket of fertility patients. Clinics will also charge extra for ICSI (which is often not actually needed) at a rate of around £1000. This makes the actual cost of one IVF treatment cycle *approximately* £8000. A more realistic estimate of the likely total costs for a single treatment cycle is £10,000 and this is a fair budget per treatment cycle. This takes into account most costs and also indirect costs such as travel and any loss of earnings related to treatment. Most patients need at least 3 treatment cycles to achieve a pregnancy making the likely total cost to be in the region of £30,000. These financial pressures are the last thing which fertility patients need but they are very real and often result in debt and increasing stress levels. I know patients who have taken out a second mortgage on their home and/or maxed out their credit cards in order to fund fertility treatment. I know of fertility patients who have spent in the region of £250,000 on fertility treatment but have had no success. There is no real answer to this problem of cost. The best advice is to ensure that the likely costs are fully understood and that they are within the budget of individual patients. This will help to reduce any big shocks in the future.

Some clinics offer 'IVF packages' and promise a 100% refund if a pregnancy is not achieved within a given time frame. The cost of such a package is around £9000 but this is subject to the usual extra fees for things such as ICSI, blood tests and medication. There are also extra costs if any additional consultations or treatments are needed beyond those available within the package. On first sight these treatment 'packages' may look attractive but often result in even more cost to the patient. For example, if patients with tubal infertility and a good sperm count take on such a package and get pregnant at the first attempt then they will have spent £9000 plus additional costs (this could be a total of around £15,000) for one treatment cycle. In this example, a pregnancy has been achieved so no refund is available. If you are considering some sort of IVF package, then please make sure that you fully understand the terms and conditions of the package. This will avoid a lot of stress and disappointment in the future. Please remember that these packages exist to make money, not to help patients.

Equally, fertility patients with complex fertility issues in both the male and the female are unlikely to qualify for 'IVF packages' because their chance of success is low. The IVF package company will therefore run a high risk of being asked to make a refund to these patients following un-successful treatment. Patients should also be aware that the refund, if payable, may only cover the basic fee charged by the fertility clinic which as described above is much lower than the actual cost. The financial side of IVF is a minefield which patients tread effectively wearing a blindfold. If fertility patients insist on transparency and clarity of information which clinics provide then this minefield can be more easily negotiated. The final solutions to this lack of transparency will be driven by patients supported by advocates such as myself.

PROFIT (OK, BUT NOT TOO MUCH!)

There is, of course, no objection to private IVF clinics making a profit on the service they provide. This applies to every private medical clinic in every medical specialism around the world. If those clinics provide an excellent and effective service to mankind, then they deserve to make a modest profit. The problem in IVF is that there is a lack of transparency about what is being offered, and the success rates and efficacy of treatment are vague. This lack of transparency results in patients not being able to see and budget for the actual cost of their treatment and being offered many expensive 'add-ons' (see Chapter 7) which are both ineffective and expensive. Fertility clinics in the UK are regulated by the HFEA for the quality and safety of the service which they provide but they are not regulated at all in terms of consumer (patient) protection. Consumer protection and rights legislation is operational in most countries, but it does not seem to apply to fertility clinics or perhaps fertility patients do not exercise their right to be treated fairly. When choosing an IVF clinic please ensure that the chosen clinic produces clear, factual and unbiased information. This will not be easy but if enough fertility patients demand transparency and truth then all fertility patients will benefit.

PUBLIC PROVISION OF IVF SERVICES (DIFFICULT TO DELIVER)

In countries such as the UK, where there is a public health service (The National Health Service, NHS) providing on-demand healthcare at the point of need free of charge, there is often a provision to provide free on-demand fertility services. Despite this, the public funding to provide this service has to come out of the same budget as that for all other publicly funded healthcare services, from family medicine to emergency treatment or surgery. This budget has to cover every aspect of healthcare in the UK. The total NHS budget in 2020 was £149 billion with an extra £63 billion to be spent on COVID-19 related expenses. In 2021, the

NHS budget will be £159 billion with an extra £22 billion spent on COVID-19 related expenses. The budgets may sound enormous (they are!) but running an on-demand, free of charge, state of the art healthcare service for a population of 68 million people is extremely expensive. There is also the fact that people are living much longer and therefore need more complex interventions and medication than what was needed in the past. The UK life-expectancy at the time of writing was at 81 years old. This means that there is an ever-increasing elderly population with an ever-increasing demand for expensive healthcare. Something has to give.

This puts enormous pressure on the healthcare service providers (in this case the NHS) who have to provide totally free healthcare for everyone from birth to death.

It can easily be seen that the problem lies in the amount of money available which can be allocated to the provision of free IVF treatment to fertility patients in need. There is a considerable demand for funding from all other areas within public healthcare and fertility services have to join the queue. Some people say that infertility is not a disease and that patients will not die (or deteriorate in any medical way) if they cannot access free treatment. The argument that infertility is not a disease is true in that, in my opinion, infertility is a *symptom* of underlying disease *e.g.* blocked tubes in the female or lack of sperm production in the male or whatever the underlying cause of infertility may be. The underlying cause of infertility is the disease. Infertility is a symptom of that disease. The question of whether or not people will die if free infertility treatment is not provided is also worth further analysis. If patients cannot access free fertility treatment, then they may well be disappointed or frustrated but their life is not in threat in the same way as a patient who has had a heart attack, a diagnosis of cancer, has suffered a stroke or has been a victim in a road accident or act of violence. Using fertility treatment as an analogy in this context does not make any sense at all and it is totally inappropriate to try to compare fertility treatment with general healthcare. Nevertheless, there have been very sad cases of suicide related to infertility but this results from poor provision of mental health and support services and not to the lack of fertility treatment. Mental health funding has in the past been poor, but improvements are being made. It is impossible to suggest that a lack of fertility treatment may lead to suicide. The whole situation is far too complex for such a claim. The events which lead to a suicide attempt may include anxiety about infertility, but infertility cannot be realistically proposed as a cause of suicide. This may sound tough to patients going through such things but it is a sad fact of life.

In the UK, there is also an IVF 'postcode lottery' in that certain areas of the country have better provision for public fertility services than others. Some private clinics have agreements with the NHS to provide fertility treatment and are paid by the NHS to deliver the service. Some large hospitals in the UK have their own IVF clinics as part of the hospital. These are often Centres of Excellence such as Guy's Hospital in London which has not only an excellent standard IVF clinic but is also a Centre of Excellence for Pre-implantation Genetic Diagnosis (PGD) technology. PGD enables the detection of genetic disease in embryos and the selection of embryos which do not carry any disease for replacement and pregnancy. This enables families who know that they carry genetic disorders to have children who do not have any disease. This is clearly a very important service which in the long-term may result in less cost to the NHS in caring for people suffering from genetic disease and of course considerably less suffering in those families where genetic disease is present.

The National Institute for Health and Health Care Excellence (NICE) recommends that infertile women in the UK under 40 years of age should be offered 3 IVF treatment cycles free of charge on the NHS. Women aged 40-42 years may be offered 1 cycle of treatment only. Some NHS clinics will only offer treatment to those women aged under 35 and may not offer treatment to patients who are obese or who are smokers.

The public provision of fertility treatment is therefore complex with many hoops through which fertility patients must jump if they are to be receive public funded fertility treatment. There is considerable debate about whether or not this situation is either desirable or ethical. What is clear is that people who can afford to pay for private fertility treatment may find it easier and less stressful to obtain treatment using that route. The outcome (live birth rate) is comparable in the public and private sectors because the technology used is the same. I have worked in both the public and private fertility sector as a Clinical Embryologist and the overall quality of service provided by both sectors is broadly the same. It is interesting to note that the first ever IVF clinic (Bourn Hall Clinic) was created as a private clinic because at that time no one in the NHS was interested in supporting IVF in any way at all. As the years have passed the NHS have recognised the importance of fertility services and introduced them in a limited fashion but the fertility treatment provision in the UK, and in the rest of the world, remains largely provided by private clinics.

The best thing for the fertility patient is to assume that free IVF treatment from a public healthcare provider of any sort may not be available. If it is available, it will be limited and it will have strict acceptance criteria. This mind-set will prevent a lot of stress and disappointment when seeking fertility treatment.

TREATMENT CYCLE NUMBERS (SIZE IS NOT EVERYTHING)

Private IVF clinics present an enormous amount of data to prospective fertility patients to get their business. Private clinic websites are packed with statistics and pictures of happy couples with their baby. This is basic marketing practice, and the private clinics cannot be blamed for presenting a rosy picture for their potential patients. Anyone who has been through IVF will know that this rosy picture may be a long way from the actual experience of IVF. Do not be fooled by clever marketing in any part of life but most importantly not in healthcare.

These private IVF clinics are by their very nature sometimes relatively small and sometimes relatively large. Small clinics may treat around 800 patients a year, larger clinic may be treating over 3,000 patients per year. Those clinics who treat 3,000 or more patients a year sometimes try to make the claim that their high throughput of patients gives them sort of edge in terms of live birth rate. This is nonsense. In fact, those fertility clinics with very high numbers of patients have an overall live birth rate just the same as those clinics with lower patient numbers. The difference in the larger clinics is that they have less time for their patients. This means that patients in high throughput clinics often feel that they are just a number and do not receive any continuity of care. My own experience is that the smaller clinics in general provide better overall patient care. If I needed fertility treatment I would go for a smaller clinic and not one of the giant 'conveyor belt' clinics.

'FAMOUS' (OR INDEED INFAMOUS) CLINIC STAFF

Another marketing ploy used by many IVF clinics is to try to suggest that some of their staff may be 'famous' and that this fame will in some way be of benefit to you as a fertility patient. You know what I am going to say to this: this is nonsense! My own experience of so called 'famous' fertility specialists is that they have an enormous ego, have little time for their patients and would much rather be giving a lecture or appearing on TV than taking time to care for their patients. Fame does not matter in any way in the delivery of first-class fertility treatment and in fact it may even be detrimental to patient care in IVF clinics. When choosing an IVF clinic do not look for fame. If an IVF clinic has 'famous' staff, then it most certainly does not mean that the 'famous' staff have any magical insight into IVF treatment or produce better live-birth rates. Possibly just the opposite. Look for caring clinic staff whose many priority is to give the best possible treatment to their patients is the best advice available here.

IVF MARKETING (CAVEAT EMPTOR!)

IVF clinics spend an enormous amount of time, energy and money on marketing their services to potential patients. Some patients will be referred to a fertility clinic by a GP or they may find themselves at a clinic which has been recommended by friends or family. The vast majority of fertility patients choose their IVF clinic based on the marketing which that clinic produces. Many clinics even attend fertility shows (there are many such shows or exhibitions now across the world) where they have a booth showing their skills and staff to potential patients. This can be an effective way of recruiting patients into a fertility clinic. The marketing from an IVF clinic will always include live-birth rate statistics as described below but there will be other things which marketeers use to capture patients. Most clinics produce pretty brochures and detailed hard copy information. Every clinic has a website where they can extol their virtues. The factual side of marketing, such as live-birth rate and treatments offered, are monitored closely by regulatory authorities. In general terms, in most countries in the world, this information is therefore as reliable as it can possibly be. The more nebulous parts of marketing such as claims that a particular clinic is 'the best' or that a particular clinic has some sort of technique, staff or knowledge which others do not is clearly meaningless. Many patients will also use patient testimonials as part of their marketing. Here the testimonial may talk about how marvellous the staff in the clinic are, how Dr. X is brilliant and how they got pregnant at the first attempt. There are two main problems with testimonials. First of all, it is impossible to know who wrote the testimonial, it could have been written by anyone from a fertility patient to a marketing man. Most likely a marketing man. Secondly, even if a testimonial is true and the treatment and outcome was perfect, then this is what is known scientifically as an anecdotal report. The means that such an experience and outcome is great for that particular patient, but it does not mean that the treatment, experience and outcome will be as good for another patient.

IVF CLINIC STATISTICS (IS THAT BLACK ACTUALLY WHITE OR IS IT GREY?)

We all know that there are lies, damned lies and statistics. My statistics lecturer in Cambridge often told me that statistics can prove anything, and they often did! The combination of IVF, enthusiastic marketing and statistics is a minefield not only for healthcare professionals but also for patients. The basic problem is that all private IVF clinics compete on their perceived success rate (live birth rate) and how this is measured and expressed is where statisticians have their most fun (if statisticians ever actually have fun). IVF clinics report a vast swathe of statistics to their respective regulatory authorities including egg collection rates, ovarian stimulation rates, fertilisation rates, embryo quality, embryo transfer rate, day 14 pregnancy rate, day 35 viable pregnancy scan rate, live birth rate and birth defect rates. These are all reported by the different age groups undergoing IVF and the result is a mass of totally incomprehensible data.

The only statistic which is of any importance at all to the patients is the live birth rate, this is after all why IVF exists and the ultimate goal of any patient. Having a fantastic fertilisation rate or 'beautiful' embryos followed by a negative pregnancy test (or worse still a positive pregnancy test and a later early miscarriage) is a failure from the point of view of the patient and that information is therefore meaningless to the patient. It is also tricky to properly record the outcome of all IVF treatment cycles in terms of live birth rate because it is 9 months before any data are available. By that time people may have moved house, or even moved Country, which often results in incomplete data! Despite this, it is possible to look back over some specific years and to create statistics which at least provide some information on live birth rate. The live birth data in the UK for example for the period from 2014 to 2016 is as follows:

29% for women under 35

23% for women aged 35-37

15% for women aged 38-39

9% for women and 40 to 42

3% for women aged 43 to 44

2% for women aged over 44

The most important thing to note from these statistics is that the age of the female patient has a considerable impact on the live birth rate. The age of the male partner does not seem to have any impact at all or if it does then it is much more subtle. These data represent nature and normal biology, no fertility clinic can change this (to my knowledge). This means that the younger the female patient comes for IVF treatment the better the likely outcome. This seems a simple way to make IVF most effective. The problem here of course is that most people do not discover that they are infertile until they try to have a family and in modern terms this is commonly not before a female age of 30-35 years. The second very striking thing which is shown by these statistics is that the live birth rate decreases considerably as the female patient approaches 40 years of age and that female patients over the age of 40 can expect fertility treatment to fail in 97-98% of attempts! These patients aged over 40 are also the patients which clinics are likely to be recommended every extra and 'add-on' (all by the way totally pointless) in the universe. These extras and 'add-ons' sadly make no difference at all to the final outcome, but they do increase the cost of the treatment considerably. We therefore have the situation where the patients least likely to succeed have treatment which costs considerably more than any other patient. There is also a considerably increased risk of Down's Syndrome in a mother aged over 40 using her own eggs which is an added complication, worry and risk in these patients.

IVF clinics will attempt to massage these data in order to produce a rosier picture or to suggest that their clinic does something differently to the others. A clinic may, for example, claim a live birth rate of 50%. When such claims are looked at more closely, then it becomes very apparent that the claim was based on a group of 10 women, all aged below 24, whose partners had perfect sperm and the cause of infertility was damaged tubes! Low patient numbers and 'easy to treat' infertility means that such claims are totally irrelevant to the average fertility patient. I have said this earlier, but I will say it again: The overall live-birth rate for IVF across all diagnoses and ages is at the very best 30%. Anyone who claims any different is either manipulating the data or is sitting on a major breakthrough and is too shy to tell anyone. I suspect the former.

SERVICE (GOOD, BAD OR INDIFFERENT)

Many IVF clinics say that they are dedicated, experienced people with their only interest being the patient (at least in their advertising). If this was true, then I would not need to write this book. This philosophy might apply to some fertility clinics, but it certainly does not apply to all. It is very difficult for someone who is considering a particular fertility clinic to decide on which clinic is the best for them. The obvious evidence may be patient testimonials, but these are of course very unreliable as described earlier. Better still if a family member or trusted friend has attended the clinic and gives their views to you personally. Failing that, talk to a fellow patient in the waiting room (this is allowed but probably not encouraged by most clinics because of what you might hear). This conversation should not be about personal treatment in any way but their general opinion of the clinic and the service they have received. These types of interactions may give you re-assurance and if not, please do not be afraid to walk away. There are plenty more IVF clinics out there!

There are a few basic things which you should expect from a private IVF clinic which are as follows:

- Attention and respect from *all staff* at *all times*.
- Staff who explain things without being patronising.
- Clear information (hard copy and electronic) on every aspect of your treatment.
- A friendly, clean environment in all areas of the clinic.

- Extra support if you need it (ideally not at an extra charge).
- The ability to fit in with your routine and a consideration of your convenience within reason.
- If you are late for an appointment for any reason the clinic should try their very best to still see you. This should be possible apart from in extreme circumstances. I have seen patients who were 10 minutes late for an appointment being turned away! This is not good service.
- Timely appointments and procedures for you (remember this is a private clinic, you are a paying customer).
- The extensive use of electronic information and support (some clinics are still largely paper based!).

    There are of course other things which you consider important, but I would suggest this list as an absolute basic requirement. If a clinic goes beyond this list, then you have found a great clinic or at least a clinic slightly better than the rest!

FERTILITY CLINIC FACILITIES

The facilities which a clinic provides to patients vary enormously. There are several clinics for example in major cities, where car parking is either extremely limited or non-existent. This may not be important until you are visiting the clinic for a scan, short of time and cannot find parking anywhere. Then it becomes extremely stressful and annoying. The appearance of a clinical may be important to some patients. I have seen clinics based in a Tudor Manor House and others on the top floor of a block of what boils down to being an industrial estate. I know which one I would choose. There are still some clinics which get very hot in the summer and very cold in the winter. A very hot treatment or scan room is a very unpleasant place to be both for staff and patients. A good IVF clinic should have air conditioning so that patients are comfortable at any time of year. Most clinics have coffee machines and water fountains available for patients and these should, of course, be free of charge to patients.

One thing which I have seen a few times over the years are clinics with no area where patients can talk to staff privately. Such conversation may be about money, the treatment itself, a complaint you may have or anything where you want privacy. This problem is most common in the reception or waiting areas of clinics where the desk and staff are often in the 'open plan' same area. Your privacy (and confidentiality) must be respected at all times and if you feel uncomfortable in any way then tell the staff.

It is arguable that a given clinic will not meet every requirement of every patient. This may be impossible because different people have different needs and expectations. Despite this, I would still suggest that the overall ambience of the clinic is important to you because it will help you to be more relaxed which in turn might even help the outcome of your treatment.

FERTILITY CLINIC STAFF

There are 4 main groups of staff in every IVF clinic. These are physicians (doctors), nurses and healthcare assistants, clinical embryologists and administration. The staff in a clinic must operate as a coherent team, if not the service provided to patients will suffer and the overall success rates might also suffer. In a good clinic all of these staff need to be well qualified. In the case of physicians this will include the usual medical degrees and very often Fellowship or Membership of a Royal College such as the Royal College of Obstetricians and Gynaecologists (F/MRCOG) in the UK. Physicians may also have research degrees such as a Ph.D. The nurses (who also supervise the health care assistants) will also have their relevant degrees and the nurses will be registered with a professional body such as the Nursing and Midwifery Council (NMC) in the UK. Most healthcare assistants will have a healthcare qualification if they do not have a degree and experience in the healthcare sector. The clinical embryologists will have their basic science degree and quiet often a research degree such as a Ph.D. All fully trained clinical embryologists in the UK must be registered with the Healthcare Professionals Council (HCPC) as Clinical Scientists (Embryology) and many will also be a Fellow or Member of the Royal College of Pathologists (F/MRCPath). The administration staff will often have degrees in business or a general degree. A degree level education is not mandatory for administration staff. These are the paper qualifications of the staff but of course there is more to being a good healthcare professional than qualifications. A good healthcare professional has understanding and empathy but also is a good listener and has complete focus on the patient. If the clinic staff are stressed or over-worked then this is bound to reflect in the quality of patient care. Finally, it is helpful if you actually like the staff in the IVF clinic. If you are going to a clinic to see people you don't like, then it may be time to change your clinic. Changing clinics is a relatively simple process in that all of your previous medical and scientific records will be sent from the old clinic to the new clinic very easily and if the clinic you want to leave claims otherwise then your next step is to seek help and advice from the regulatory authority which is the HFEA in the UK.

FERTILITY CLINIC TECHNOLOGY

The technology available in an IVF clinic may be presented to you by the clinic as being bigger, better or more effective than anyone else. If you see or hear such a claim from an IVF clinic in their marketing, or indeed anywhere else, then I would suggest walking away. The technology currently used to provide IVF is pretty much standardised and no one really has bigger or better. The equipment is what it is. The ultrasound scanners used to monitor follicular growth and to assess ongoing pregnancies are available from several manufacturers, but they all broadly do the same job. Some may offer slight innovations or extra data available, but this should not be used as a selling point for the clinic. The equipment in the operating theatre where all surgical procedures take place is equally standardised and no one really has the edge in this area.

The embryology laboratory is potentially the place where the greatest variation of equipment manufacturers and suppliers may be found but once again the different manufacturers and suppliers offer pretty much the same level of service so claiming that one piece of equipment has some sort of edge or benefit on another does not really work. In the early days of IVF possibly the biggest potential technical variation in the laboratory was the culture medium in which the embryos grow. This was because the media were prepared 'in house' by the clinical embryologists. Today all clinics use clinically approved (CE marked) media and consumables produced by fully accredited manufacturers so there can be no claims of superiority from different manufacturers. The problem with this of course is that media and consumables produced to such stringent specification are expensive and this cost is passed on to the patients. The regulatory authorities have been extremely helpful in standardising what an IVF clinic can and cannot do which means that any licensed IVF clinic is operating to the optimum standards of quality and safety. It is also useful to note that all IVF clinics want their clinic to have the best possible live-birth rate for marketing purposes. This means that the 'best' equipment and reagents often naturally find their way into all clinics as no clinic will use anything which is either unlicensed or performs poorly. If they did then this would affect their license status and also potentially their live-birth rate.

QUESTIONS TO ASK A FERTILITY CLINIC

Some regulatory authorities, such as the HFEA in the UK (the link is in the useful links section at the end of this book), are starting to provide potential patients with a list of approved questions which patients should ask at their first consultation at a fertility clinic. This is a very welcome innovation because it begins to empower fertility patients in what can seem a very daunting and even threatening atmosphere. I would suggest that all fertility patients should arm themselves with these questions and if you get poor replies, then say so and ask for a better opinion or reply from someone else in the clinic. These questions, and the replies, you receive could save a lot of time, money and stress and may even help you to choose the best and most successful fertility clinic for you.

KEY POINTS OF CHAPTER 5

- Private fertility clinics primarily exist to make money.
- Fertility treatment may be available in the public sector, but it may not.
- A very large and 'famous' clinic is not always the best clinic.
- IVF clinic statistics should be viewed with a healthy scepticism unless they are reported by a regulatory authority.
- Fertility clinic staff and facilities will vary enormously. Choose a clinic and staff which you like and feel confident about, this is a personal judgement.
- Remember that in a private fertility clinic you are a fee-paying customer, and your consumer rights apply.
- Fertility clinic technology is pretty standard, do not be 'blinded by science'.
- Arm yourself with regulatory authority approved questions for your first consultation.

CHAPTER 6

The Basic Treatment

Peter Hollands

(Current IVF Technology)

> *Adopt the pace of nature: her secret is patience.*
> **Ralph Waldo Emerson**

Summary: This chapter describes the actual process of IVF from the point of view of the patient and also from a 'behind the scenes' viewpoint where relevant. This may be very useful for patients who are new to IVF and it might even be helpful to those patients who are undergoing or have undergone treatment. There may be slight variations from clinic to clinic, but the basic principles should apply to all clinics.

INTRODUCTION

A fertility treatment cycle is a daunting and even frightening process for some people. If there are aspects of your treatment which frighten or worry you, then please do not hesitate to speak to your fertility clinic staff for help, support, information and re-assurance. Such concerns may be amplified for 'first-time' patients, but they may occur in all patients at any time. Please also remember that your clinic has an excellent independent counsellor available to speak to you and this can be a priceless resource for some patients. The main piece of advice is to listen very carefully to what the fertility clinic staff tell you about your treatment and if you are unsure or do not understand anything, then ask them to explain it again. Your total understanding of what your treatment will involve and what you have to do during that treatment is critical to success.

THE FERTILITY MEDICATIONS

There are many medications which the female patient has to take during an IVF treatment cycle. The first thing to clearly understand is that all of these medications add-up to a significant cost to the patient above the basic quote for treatment. The IVF clinic should make this very clear to you but please do not get caught out by this, it is a very significant cost. The medication will be all self-administered following detailed instructions and tuition from the nurses in the IVF clinic. The IVF treatment cycle starts at the beginning of menstruation of the female. The first drug used in most treatment cycles is called Suprefact (generic name Buserelin) or an identical drug from another manufacturer. This drug is most often taken by sniffing it into the nose, but it can also be given by injection. The purpose of this medication is to suppress (technically known as down-regulation) the natural cycle so that all reproductive hormones fall down to zero. This effectively gives a 'blank page' on which the treatment cycle will be based.

The next basic medication is a drug which stimulates the growth of follicles in the ovary. The technical term for these drugs is 'gonadotrophins' (known as gonadotropins in some countries). These are usually injected daily into the fat around the abdominal area and typical examples are Gonal F, Follistim and many more. These are usually the most expensive medications in a fertility treatment cycle, and some patients will need more of this medication than others, depending on the response of the ovaries. The next medication is used when the follicular development is at the optimum stage is Profasi which is known generically as human chorionic gonadotrphin (hCG). This injection ensures that the egg will be in an optimal condition at the time of egg collection and is often known as the 'trigger'. The time from trigger (or hCG) injection to egg collection is usually around 36 hours and this timing is ***very important*** to ensure optimal quality eggs are collected and to ensure that uncontrolled ovulation does not take place, and the eggs are lost. Some patients struggle with this concept that the 'trigger' must be given at a specific time, but it is a critical part of a successful treatment cycle. You will be told the time at which the 'trigger' injection must be given, and you should administer the 'trigger' injection at that time. If you miss the time for any reason, then please contact your clinic urgently for further advice. The final basic medication is a progesterone preparation which can either be injected (the most common medication used is Gestone) or taken by vaginal pessaries (the most common medication used is Cyclogest). There are other formulations which other clinics may use. Progesterone is usually taken every day from embryo replacement to pregnancy test and if pregnant, it is often continued every day until the end of the first trimester of pregnancy. If the injected form of progesterone is prescribed, then this may result in some discomfort, especially if you have to take it for a long time. If this becomes a problem, please discuss it with your clinic.

These are the basic medications used in IVF, but your clinic may use different types or preparations in different combinations. The basic principles are always the same: Down-regulate, stimulate ovaries, trigger (hCG) and supplement progesterone. There are many different stimulation protocols, and the decision on which protocol is to be used is taken by a physician. The ovarian stimulation and medication protocol will be described to you in great detail and some clinics even use phone apps to remind patients when and how to take medication. It is absolutely essential to the success of your treatment that the medication is taken correctly and at the right time. If you are unsure in any way, then please do not hesitate to ask your clinic staff for clarification.

FOLLICULAR GROWTH MONITORING

During the period of ovarian stimulation in the treatment cycle, it is important to monitor the size and number of follicles developing in each ovary. This is achieved by using a vaginal ultrasound scan which may be carried out between 5-10 times during the ovarian stimulation stage of treatment. Each scan takes 15-20 minutes, and the scan is carried out at the IVF clinic, usually by the fertility nurses. The results of the scan are reviewed by a physician who will decide the next steps. These next steps may be to reduce medication, keep medication the same, increase the medication or take the trigger (hCG) injection at the prescribed time. The fertility nurses will be able to help to explain the changes if needed, and do not be afraid to ask questions if you are unsure about anything at this stage of your treatment.

OVARIAN HYPER-STIMULATION SYNDROME

Some patients may respond too strongly to even low levels of ovarian stimulation and this can result in a condition called Ovarian Hyper-Stimulation Syndrome (OHSS). This will be detected very easily during the ultrasound scan monitoring and all clinics have clear protocols on how to manage OHSS. There will be far too many follicles developing on each ovary, and this results in problems with general body fluid balance. Sometimes OHSS can be controlled by simply increasing fluid intake (drinking plenty of water), but in a minority of patients OHSS may be so severe that hospital admission is needed in order to safely manage the syndrome. There have been very rare deaths due to OHSS but with proper monitoring and management, it should be possible to control the syndrome. Patients who suffer OHSS are often advised to freeze all of the embryos which develop for replacement in another cycle. This is a routine precaution and something which protects the health of the female patient because a pregnancy as well as OHSS may be very difficult to safely handle.

THE EGG COLLECTION

Following the administration of hCG, at the correct time, you will be given the time of your egg collection at the clinic. These typically start at about 8.30 am in most clinics and continue until all egg collections for that day have been completed. In a busy clinic, this may be early to mid-afternoon. Each egg collection takes about 20-30 minutes, assuming that there are no complications such as bleeding. When you both arrive at the clinic, the female partner, or the partner to undergo egg collection, will be checked for general health and clinical parameters such as blood pressure and temperature. The female will also have a quick talk with the anaesthetist who will be administering the sedation for the egg collection procedure. This will include such things as any allergies that the patient may have and any respiratory problems she may have. The anaesthetist will be able to answer any questions you may have. The female then goes to the theatre, and the sedation is administered. This is not a general anaesthetic, but you will not remember anything about the procedure, and you will not feel any pain during the procedure.

The eggs are collected by using a vaginal ultrasound probe to direct the collection needle to each separate follicle in the ovary. The contents of the follicle are gently sucked into a collection pot and this is then handed to the laboratory to check to see if an egg is present. If the egg is present, then the surgeon then moves onto the next follicle and so on until all of the follicles have been drained and the eggs collected. Sometimes an egg is not found in every follicle and the surgeon makes the decision to move on to a fresh follicle if an egg has not been found. The human egg is about 0.1mm in diameter and it is surrounded by cells called granulosa cells which support and 'feed' the egg during development. The whole structure is therefore just visible by the naked eye, but embryologists use a low power microscope in the laboratory in order to quickly and properly find the eggs.

Following the egg collection, the female partner is taken to the recovery area where her vital signs (blood pressure and temperature) will be monitored during the recovery period and she will be monitored for any bleeding or any other potential problems. The female patient will be allowed to leave the clinic when the medical staff is satisfied that she has properly recovered from the procedure. Mild pain killers such as paracetamol might be needed in the period immediately following the egg collection and the fertility clinic staff are always available 'on call' if needed.

SEMEN PRODUCTION AND INSEMINATION

On the day of egg collection, the male partner has to produce a semen sample by masturbation so that the embryologists can prepare sperm to inseminate the eggs. The embryologist will provide the semen collection pot to the male patient and will discreetly escort him to the 'men's room' which is usually a private room in a quiet part of the clinic. The embryologist will check the identity of the male patient and give any specific instructions which may be needed. Following semen production, there is usually some sort of hatch into which the semen collection pot is placed (the hatch often links directly to the laboratory) and often a buzzer for the male patient to press, which alerts the laboratory (no one else!) that there is a semen sample ready to be processed. This process can be quite stressful for some male patients, especially as his partner will be in the operating theatre at this time, but if this is the case, then the male partner should discuss this with the clinic staff as it may be possible to reassure and resolve any worries before the day of egg collection.

On receipt into the laboratory, the semen sample is initially incubated for about 30 minutes to allow a process called liquefaction (a change from a viscous fluid to a less viscous fluid) to take place. Once liquified the semen can we washed with culture media and the sperm are then concentrated in preparation for insemination of the eggs.

There are two ways in which insemination is carried out and these are 'standard' IVF and Intra-Cytoplasmic Sperm Injection (ICSI). In standard IVF the eggs and sperm are simply mixed together, and natural fertilisation takes place. This can be used for all patients as long as there are sufficient sperm numbers in the sperm preparation. If there are insufficient sperm numbers for IVF, then ICSI will be used to achieve fertilisation. In this process, a single sperm is directly injected into each egg using very accurate and sensitive micromanipulation technology. There is often an additional charge for ICSI because of the expensive technology needed to provide this service.

IVF FROM A LABORATORY VIEWPOINT

There is a considerable amount of 'behind the scenes' activity in an IVF clinic which the patients do not see and it is the IVF laboratory where most of this 'behind the scenes' activity takes place. The laboratory is at the heart of IVF treatment because it is here where the quality of the embryos is defined. The laboratory is part of the treatment process from when a patient first comes to a fertility clinic to when they leave, hopefully carrying a baby! The first interaction if often the semen analysis of the male partner at the first consultation and this is when he may first meet the clinical embryologists in the clinic. This semen analysis from the IVF laboratory, along with any investigations which the female partner needs to undergo, will enable the physicians to come to a diagnosis for the cause of infertility and to create a treatment plan.

The IVF laboratory is a complex facility which is almost always attached to the operating theatre. This enables the easy transfer of eggs to the laboratory at egg collection and to return the embryos to the patient at embryo replacement. The laboratory and the clinic operate under the regulatory body license (the HFEA in the UK), which means that the laboratory and staff must adhere to strict levels of quality, reproducibility, safety and traceability to ensure that the safety and quality of the service to patients is optimised. The laboratory must use equipment and consumables which have been approved for clinical use and the staff must all be properly trained and competent and where required, registered with the appropriate professional body such as the HCPC in the UK.

At egg collection the laboratory will have prepared carefully labelled 'dishes' which contain drops of culture media under liquid paraffin. The eggs which are collected will be placed into these drops of media and they will be stored in this way for a few hours before insemination. The insemination will be carried out as described above and the inseminated eggs are then left in the incubator overnight. The following morning an embryologist will check each egg under the microscope to see if it has been fertilised. This can be seen by the appearance of two small spots in the egg called pronuclei which are the male and female DNA coming together ready to produce a new embryo. The fertilisation at this stage is usually reported to the patients by the embryologists so that they are well informed about the progress of their treatment. There is, of course, the possibility that none of the eggs have fertilised and if so, this is reported to the patients and arrangements are made for a follow-up consultation and for any support which the patients may need.

Assuming good fertilisation the embryos are then kept in the incubator in the laboratory for up to 5 days (to a stage called a blastocyst) counting the day of egg collection as Day 0. Most IVF clinics now replace embryos at what is known as the blastocyst stage. A blastocyst is a hollow ball of around 120 cells. There is a thicker area on the ball of cells called the inner cell mass (ICM) and this will develop into the fetus. The thinner cells of the ball are called the trophoblast and these cells will develop into the placenta and the membranes which eventually surround the baby. The blastocyst is the embryonic stage just before implantation into the uterus. Some clinics may replace embryos on day 3 of development which is usually a 8-12 cell embryo. These embryos then grow in the uterus to the blastocyst stage and are then implant into the uterus.

On the day of embryo replacement, the laboratory prepares all of the equipment and reagents needed and the actual embryo replacement procedure is described below. In the laboratory, it is a matter of choosing the best embryo to replace (most clinics replace one embryo to minimise multiple pregnancies) and loading it into a very soft catheter. This is then handed to the surgeon, who inserts the catheter into the uterus through the cervix and places the embryo on the perfect spot to implant.

As each woman produces several eggs during IVF there is almost always some 'spare' embryos at the end of the process. If these 'spare' embryos are of good quality, then they can be frozen for later use if the patient does not become pregnant or for future treatments without the need for an egg collection. The laboratory also stores frozen sperm when needed which can either be from the male partner or from a donor sperm bank. Some clinics also store frozen donor eggs for use by patients if needed.

THE EMBRYO REPLACEMENT (TRANSFER)

On the day of embryo replacement, the couple are both invited back to the clinic at the correct time. It is good if the male partner can attend the replacement process to support his partner and also to feel part of the process. On arrival, there will be the usual identity checks and the female partner will be asked to change into a gown in preparation for the embryo replacement. The male partner is usually asked to put a gown over his outdoor clothes and might also get a very nice hat to wear!

Once in theatre a seat is given to the male (next to his partner) and the female partner is positioned on the bed in readiness for the embryo replacement. The embryologist then talks to the patients about the embryo which is going to be replaced and answers any questions they might have. At this stage almost all IVF clinics have a monitor in the theatre on which can be seen the embryo chosen for replacement, most clinics can also give the patients a photograph of the embryo replaced. This is in general a good thing, although I have heard of patients whose treatment failed giving perhaps too much attention for too long to the photo of their embryo. If you find yourself grieving for your embryo from a failed treatment cycle, then please ask for support from your fertility clinic.

The replacement procedure itself is similar to a cervical smear procedure. This surgeon will insert an instrument into the vagina which allows the visualisation of the cervix. The embryologist loads the embryo for replacement into a very soft catheter and hands this to the surgeon. The surgeon then passes the catheter through the cervix with ultrasound guidance and places the embryo in the perfect spot. The patients then go the recovery area for a short while and they are then free to go home.

Patients often worry that embryos will 'fall out' but this is not the case. In the early days of IVF, patients were kept lying down for up to one hour after embryo replacement. More recent experience has shown that this is not necessary or beneficial in any way. Patients also often ask if there is anything they should do following embryo replacement, but the best answer is to go back to normal life as long as normal life does not include daily marathon running! It is a good idea to take some sort of break or holiday following embryo replacement to relax while waiting for the pregnancy test.

EMBRYO FREEZING AND REPLACEMENT

On the day of embryo replacement, the clinical embryologists will assess the remaining embryos for possible freezing. This decision is based on the appearance and rate of growth of the remaining embryos, and you will be told how many (if any) embryos are suitable for freezing during the replacement procedure. The purpose of embryo freezing is to enable their use later as a source of embryos without the need for a further full treatment cycle. The procedure is either called a Frozen Embryo Replacement (FER) or Frozen Embryo Transfer (FET). If your fresh treatment cycle was a success, then the frozen embryos represent a source of possible siblings for your baby.

The embryos are frozen in liquid nitrogen (usually at the blastocyst stage) at a temperature of -196°C. Your clinic will charge you an additional fee for the freezing process and also an annual fee for the ongoing storage of your embryos. At the temperature of liquid nitrogen, the frozen embryos are in theory stable forever. Despite this the regulatory authorities place a maximum limit on storage times of 10 years on most embryos. This time is usually plenty to allow the use of the frozen embryos by the patients. Extended storage can be agreed in some cases, especially if there are medical reasons for extended storage.

Some frozen embryos will not be needed by the patients and in this case the frozen embryos can be discarded or sometimes donated to research. This is a very careful procedure which begins with detailed discussions with the parents followed by written authority for the embryos to either be discarded or donated to research. If the embryos are discarded, then the embryos are simply allowed to thaw and discarded in the medical waste of the clinic. If the embryos are donated to research, they are often sent to a research laboratory where they will be used for research under very strict guidelines and ethical requirements. Human embryos may also be used to produce human embryonic stem cells to be used in regeneration medicine procedures. This is not a common fate of frozen embryos, but it is one possibility which you may be asked to approve.

If you decide to use frozen embryos to try to achieve a pregnancy, then you will receive detailed instructions from your fertility clinic about the medication you need to take prior to the frozen embryo replacement and any other things you need to do. On the day of the frozen embryo replacement, you will be invited to attend the clinic at a given time and the replacement process and aftercare will be the same as that for a fresh embryo replacement. One word of caution is that when embryos are thawed, some embryos will not survive the thawing process. This does not mean that any mistakes or errors have taken place; it simply reflects the relatively traumatic process of freezing human cells in liquid nitrogen and then thawing them out. This means that it is possible that you may prepare for a frozen embryo replacement but on the day, there will be no embryos available for replacement. This is a relatively rare situation, but it is something you should be aware of and ready to deal with should it occur. Please also remember that you will be charged for the frozen embryo replacement (even if the embryos fail to thaw) but this charge should be considerably less than the cost of a fresh treatment cycle.

THE PREGNANCY TEST AND THE DAY 35 SCAN

Arguably the most stressful phase of fertility treatment process is the time from embryo replacement to pregnancy test. This test is usually carried out on Day 14, when Day 0 was the day of egg collection. Most clinics now ask patients to carry out the pregnancy test using an 'over the counter' testing kit from a chemist or pharmacist. Some patients cannot wait and start testing every day following embryo replacement. This is a bad idea because these early tests will just come back as negative, which only increases the stress levels. Some may even come back false positive because of medication still in remaining in your body following treatment. The best approach is to relax and try to put the pregnancy test out of your mind. This is easier said than done but in the long term, it will be better for your sanity and might even be better for the outcome of the treatment. This period is often known as the 'two-week-wait' by patients and if you can do the two-week-wait with a minimum of anxiety and stress then this is a good thing. It might even be a great time for a short break or holiday to take your mind off things.

If the pregnancy test is positive, then the clinic will ask you to begin taking folic acid (this helps to prevent the incidence of spina bifida in the developing baby and is taken by all pregnant women) and arrange for an ultrasound scan usually at around day 35. This scan will confirm a viable pregnancy (a visible fetus and a heartbeat) and from this stage the pregnant woman will be managed in exactly the same way as a natural conception. The scan may of course show an unviable pregnancy on day 35 (no heartbeat or abnormal development) and you should be prepared for this news to minimise stress. If this is the case, then the clinic will advise you on the next steps which may involve a 'D&C' in your local hospital to remove the unviable pregnancy.

If the pregnancy test is negative, then the clinic will arrange for a follow-up consultation where advice will be available on possible next steps, including another treatment cycle. Most clinics try to avoid 'back-to-back' treatment cycles as it is a good idea to give your mind and body a rest between treatment cycles.

A 'PRECIOUS' PREGNANCY

If a pregnancy resulted from an IVF treatment cycle in the early days, then the pregnancy was often regarded as 'precious'. This meant that the patient would undergo more checks during the pregnancy and a Caesarian section may be used to deliver the baby rather than a natural vaginal delivery. This approach is arguably more stressful for the patient because she may feel that either something is wrong or that something may go wrong. Today, fortunately, this idea has pretty much disappeared and women who are pregnant from an IVF treatment cycle receive the same maternity care as all other women with their GP, antenatal clinic and delivery unit. This is how it should be, once pregnant there is no difference between an IVF pregnancy and a natural pregnancy.

DONOR GAMETES (DONOR SPERM AND DONOR EGGS)

Donor Sperm

Donor sperm has been part of fertility treatment for long before IVF became routine. The first recorded case of donor sperm insemination was in 1884 and in 1945 Mary Barton published the first record of donor insemination in the UK. Sperm donors were initially anonymous, and the donor was selected for a recipient patient purely by physical characteristics such as race, height, build, complexion and eye and colour. More recently sperm donors in most countries are no longer anonymous and those children born from donor sperm can get access to the details of the sperm donor when they are adults if they choose to do so. Some people claimed that this lack of donor anonymity may reduce the number of sperm donors coming forward to donate, but it seems that this has not been the case.

Sperm donation and the use of donor sperm in fertility treatment are regulated by the same organisations which regulate IVF, *e.g.*, in the UK, the HFEA. Donors have to undergo medical examination, provide a medical history, provide blood samples for infectious disease screening and, of course, have their semen analysed to ensure that they are producing sufficient sperm numbers to potentially create a pregnancy. Assuming that all of these hurdles are passed then the donor provides semen samples for freezing. This is commonly up to around 6 different donations which are processed and frozen in liquid nitrogen.

Most countries have limits on how many families one single sperm or egg donor may be used to create. In the UK, this is currently a maximum of 10 different families from one donor. The reason for this is to reduce the chance of stepsiblings meeting and reproducing.

Donor Sperm in IVF

In the early days of IVF, donor sperm was used very often for those patients where the male produced insufficient numbers of sperm for IVF. This was before the days of ICSI and surgical sperm collections which today mean that it is fairly rare to need donor sperm for IVF patients. The exception to this is, of course, if the male patient does not produce any sperm at all and no sperm can be obtained surgically, then donor sperm is the only option. More recently, donor sperm has been used to create a pregnancy in single women, women with a totally infertile male partner and same sex female couples. Donor sperm is obtained from licensed and accredited sperm banks, which first became operational in 1970. These sperm banks recruit sperm donors (quite often these are University students) to provide the sperm for treatment. There is even one sperm bank who claims to have sperm from Nobel prize winners! The patients can find out a lot about the sperm donor in terms of build, race, complexion, infection and genetic screening, eye and hair colour and quite often a short, written piece from the donor about his motivation for donation and giving best wishes to the patients who will use the donor sperm.

Donor Eggs in IVF

Donor eggs were first used in 1983 and there have been around 50,000 pregnancies and births using donor eggs to date. Egg donors are usually recruited by specialised companies or sometimes fertility clinics themselves. They are screened for infectious diseases and undergo a thorough selection process, including medical history and medical examination. Donor eggs are most commonly used when the female patient either cannot produce eggs from her ovaries (for example, close to or after the time of menopause) and also at any age when the female patient is unable to produce eggs for any reason. Egg donors receive payment for their donation but in the UK and most other countries that payment is restricted and can only be used for reimbursement of expenses incurred by the egg donor and associated with the egg donation. Egg donation is medically more complex than sperm donation because egg collection is a surgical procedure. The details of the egg donor will be made available to the prospective parents.

KEY POINTS OF CHAPTER 6

- Fertility treatment needs specific medications which must be self-administered in the correct dose and time.
- The fertility treatment process includes egg collection, sperm collection, fertilisation in the laboratory, growth of the embryos, embryo replacement and if possible, embryo freezing.
- The two-week-wait for a pregnancy test may be stressful and the best advice is

to relax as much as possible.
- The day 35 ultrasound scan will confirm a viable pregnancy. If the pregnancy is not viable at this point, then the fertility clinic will advise you accordingly.
- Both donor sperm and donor eggs are regularly used in modern fertility treatments.

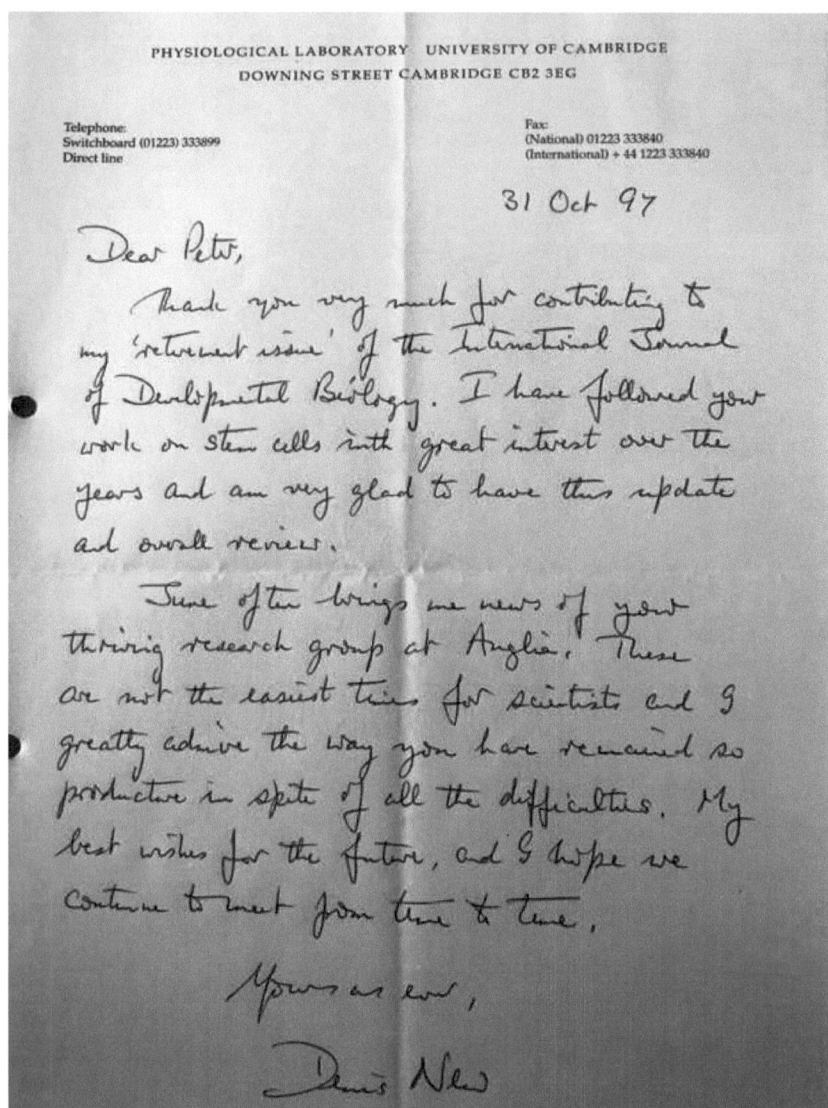

PHYSIOLOGICAL LABORATORY   UNIVERSITY OF CAMBRIDGE
DOWNING STREET CAMBRIDGE CB2 3EG

Telephone:
Switchboard (01223) 333899
Direct line

Fax:
(National) 01223 333840
(International) + 44 1223 333840

31 Oct 97

Dear Peter,

Thank you very much for contributing to my 'retirement issue' of the International Journal of Developmental Biology. I have followed your work on stem cells with great interest over the years and am very glad to have this update and overall review.

June often brings me news of your thriving research group at Anglia. These are not the easiest times for scientists and I greatly admire the way you have remained so productive in spite of all the difficulties. My best wishes for the future, and I hope we continue to meet from time to time.

Yours as ever,

Denis New

This is a letter from my dear friend and colleague Denis New thanking me for a paper I wrote to commemorate his retirement. Denis was a colleague of Bob Edwards and we often had many interesting discussions about embryos, IVF and stem cells.

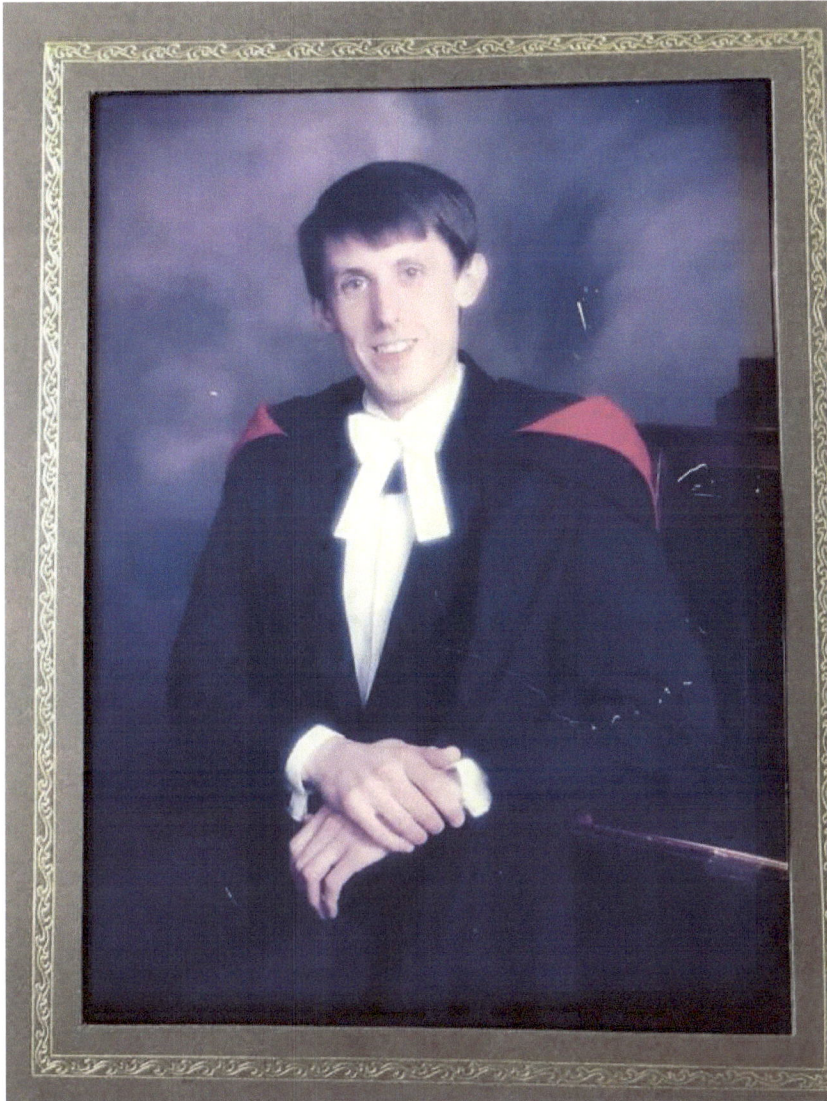

This rather scratched picture is of me on the day my PhD from Cambridge University was awarded. My research, under the supervision of Bob Edwards, focussed on the possibility of using stem cells obtained from early mouse embryos to repair damaged bone in fully grown mice. This was at the very start of Regenerative Medicine and the start of a very interesting time for me.

Embryos: the case for research

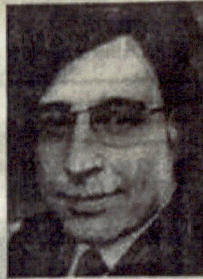

Nicholas Timmins

This is an interesting article from The Times July 1984 about human embryo research. We were always clear that human embryo research must be focussed, ethical and most of all regulated. This was a time of great debate on the subject and it resulted in the guidance and regulation on human embryo research which we all follow today.

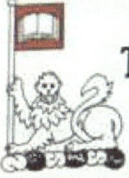

The Master & Fellows of Churchill College

Invite you to a celebration
of the award to Professor Robert Edwards
of the 2010 Nobel Prize in Physiology or Medicine

On Saturday 30 April 2011
Churchill College, Cambridge

Programme of Events

5.00 pm A programme of talks by former colleagues
and a short video presentation in the Wolfson Hall

6.30 pm Buffet reception in the Jock Colville Hall

RSVP by Friday 22 April

Rosemary Saunders
Master's PA
rosemary.saunders@chu.cam.ac.uk
01223 336142

This is an invitation to me from the Master of Churchill College, Cambridge to attend a ceremony celebrating the award of Nobel Prize in Physiology or Medicine to Bob Edwards. This was a bitter-sweet event as Bob was suffering very badly from dementia at this time, but his wife Ruth attended along with many other past colleagues and it was a memorable event.

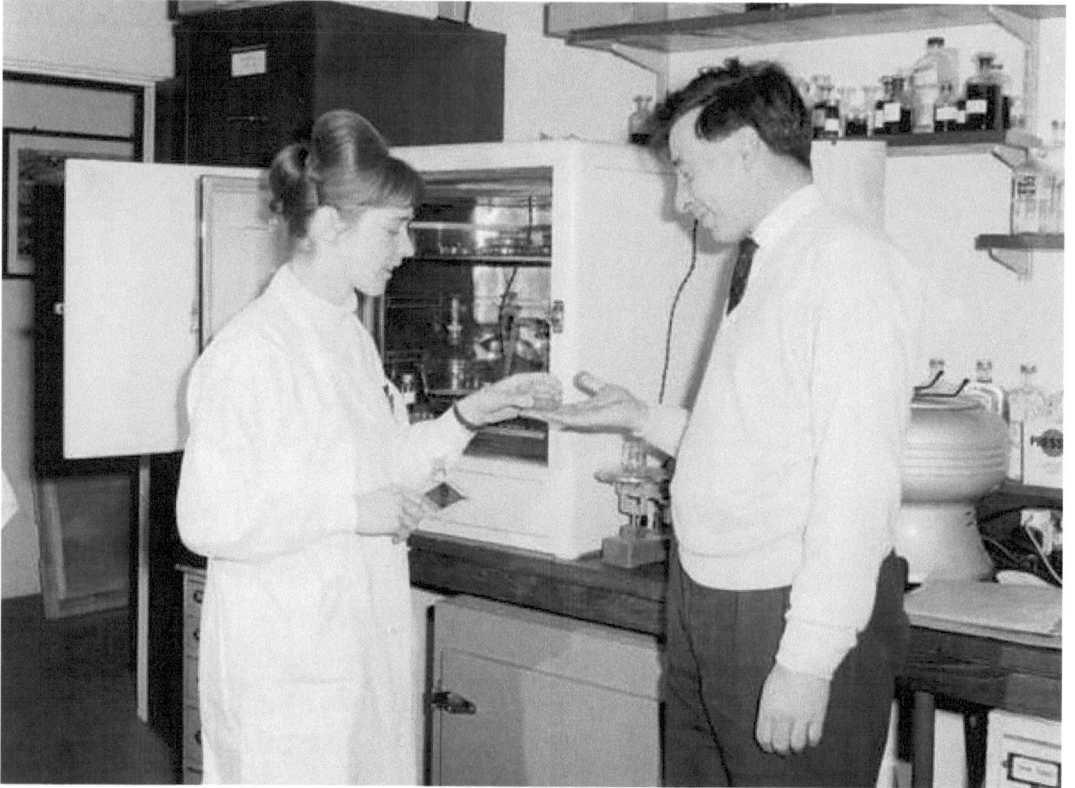

This is Jean Purdy (on the left) and Bob Edwards (on the right) in their research Laboratory in Cambridge University in 1968. In the background can be seen the type of incubator used in early IVF and it contains a glass 'gas jar' in which the human embryos were first cultured.

19 March 1985

Dr Klaus Diedrich
Department of Gynecology & Obstetrics
University of Bonn
Sigmund Frued Str. 25
D-5300 Bonn-Venusberg
FRG

Dear Klaus

I have had a very nice letter from Richard Marrs. Will
you send him details of the Society and a membership form.

I wish to submit another abstract for the Bonn meeting on
the session on in vitro fertilization. This will be given
by Peter Hollands and the lecture will be entitled
"Differentiation of Stem Cells in the Mouse Embryo and
Their Use in Grafting". Peter works here with me.

With best wishes

Yours sincerely

R G Edwards

Enc

This was a letter from Bob Edwards to Klaus Diedrich, the organiser of the first ESHRE meeting, asking him to accept a presentation from me on my PhD research on mouse embryo stem cells.

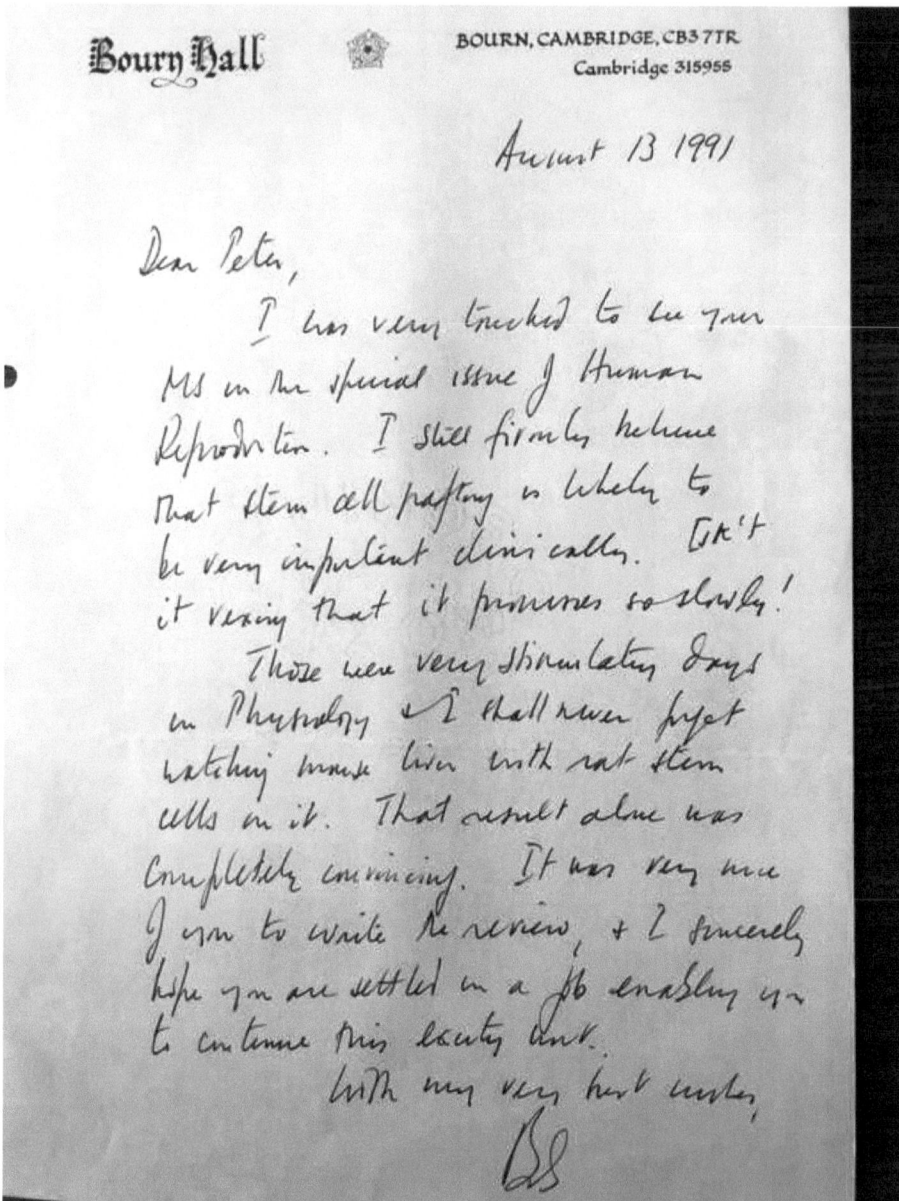

This is a letter to me from Bob Edwards about a paper I wrote for his journal Human Reproduction. He also reflects on the slow progress of stem cell technology and refers to an astonishing experiment grafting mouse cells into rats which he enabled me to do at Cambridge University. These were the first faltering steps towards regenerative medicine.

TEL. CRAFTS HILL 780602

DUCK END FARM
PARK LANE
DRY DRAYTON
CAMBRIDGE CB3 8DB

March 15 1992

Dear Peter

I'm delighted you have a chance to get back to your research in a good position. There has been too long a delay in it, such a pity. Still, you can now get back to it + I hope very successfully.

I left Bourn last year but still edit Human Reproduction from there. All the hard science seems to have left the place!

Best wishes

This is a letter to me from Bob Edwards after he had left Bourn Hall Clinic. He also reflects on the people on the original team (including me) who had left Bourn Hall Clinic. These were sad times for us all.

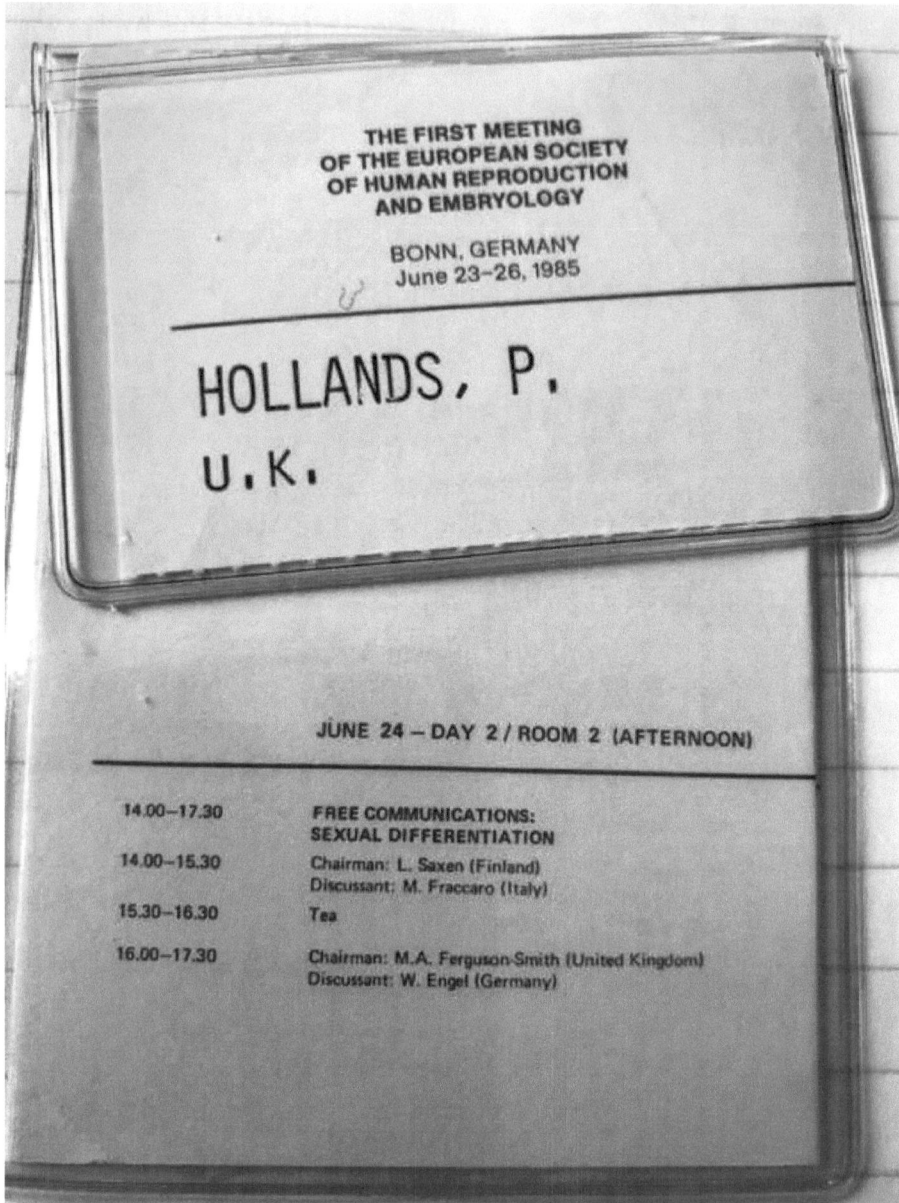

This was my identification badge for the first meeting of the European Society of Human Reproduction and Embryology on June 23-26th 1985. This was a small meeting, no more than 150 people in total, and I presented some research data from my PhD. Today this meeting has thousands of delegates and it is attended by people from around the world to hear the latest ideas in IVF.

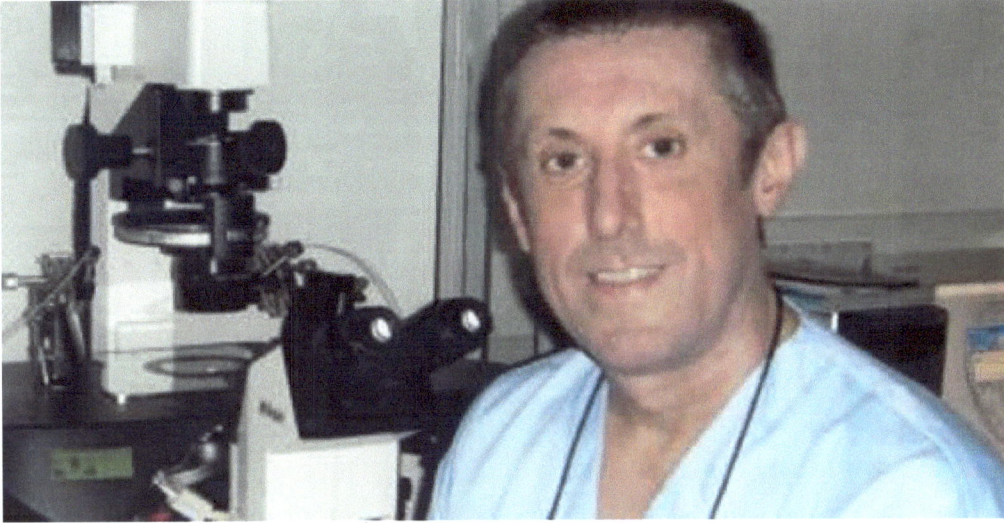

This is me in The Bridge IVF Clinic in Lagos, Nigeria. I worked as Scientific Director there and it was a great pleasure to work with Nigerian colleagues in the delivery of fertility services. The equipment in the background is known as an 'ICSI rig' which is a high power microscope and manipulators used to carry out ICSI.

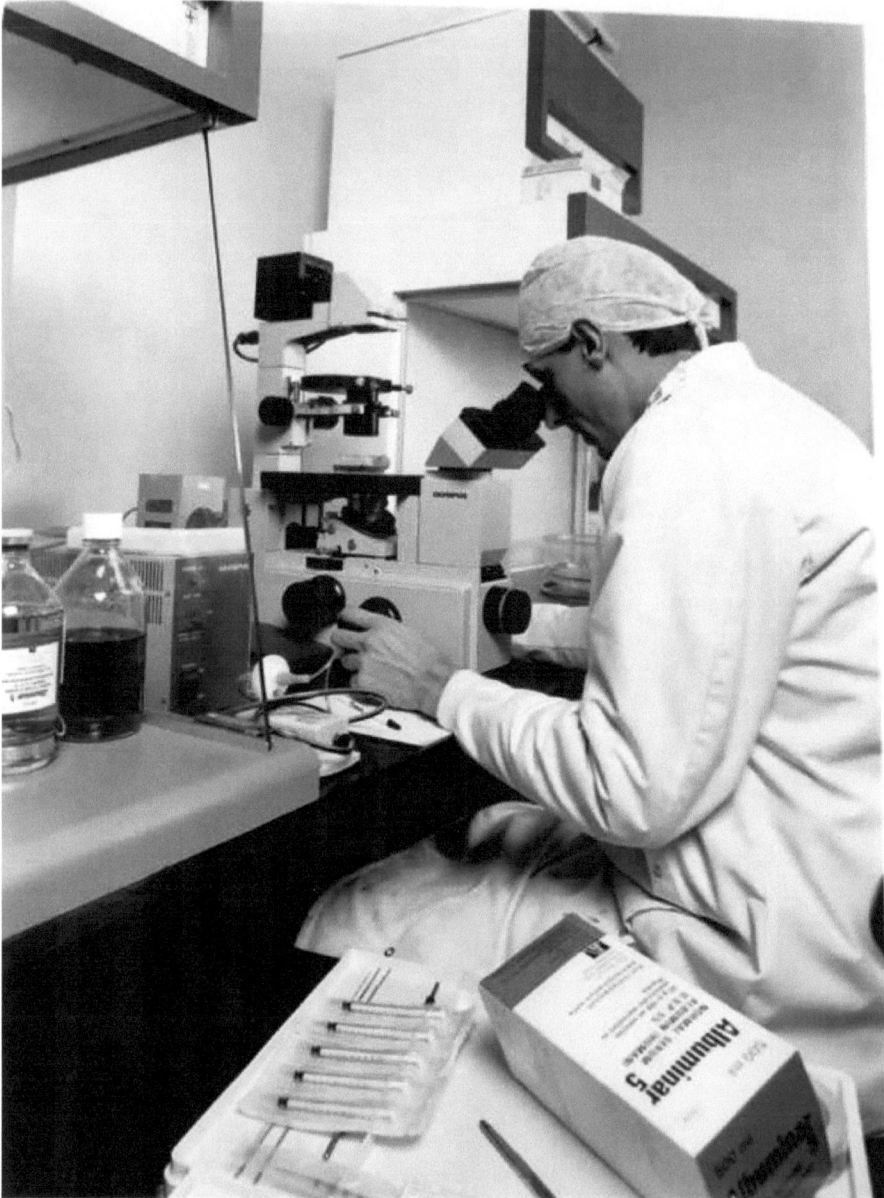

This is me in my research laboratory in Cambridge in the early 1990's. At this time I was working on umbilical cord blood stem cells and I went on to work on many different stem cell types but surprisingly enough never embryonic stem cells.

CHAPTER 7

The 'Add-Ons' Scandal

Peter Hollands

(The Use of Untested and Unproven Technology on Fertility Patients)

'Rather than love, than money, than fame, give me truth'.
Henry David Thoreau (1817-1862)

Summary: This chapter explores the murky field of IVF 'add-ons' which are offered to patients as a proposed technology to improve the overall success rate of IVF treatment. The cost of these 'add-ons' can be very high. This is a very poor situation where some fertility clinics are offering untested and unproven 'treatments' to their patients. The regulatory authorities are slowly clamping down on this practice but at the time of writing it was still a major problem in fertility clinics.

INTRODUCTION

'Add-ons' are processes and procedures which are often offered to fertility patients at additional cost to their standard treatment. The claim is that these 'add-ons' may increase the chance of success in an IVF treatment cycle. Sadly, there is no convincing evidence that 'add-ons' make any difference at all to fertility treatment success rates but what they definitely do achieve is to boost the income and profits for IVF clinics.

As I described earlier in this book, it is over 40 years since the first IVF baby was born and IVF is now a common-place medical treatment. This routine application of IVF is the culmination of decades of scientific and medical research, and the technology, whilst still far from perfect, is tried and tested. This research enabled scientists to understand how to safely bring together human eggs and sperm in the laboratory, resulting in a human embryo, which subsequently has the potential to form a healthy normal human being. There have been over 8 million IVF babies born globally but despite this, there is clearly a stagnation or even a downward trend of the IVF live birth rates. This has not stopped the financial development of IVF, with mergers and acquisitions of clinics and IVF related suppliers generating enormous amounts of money in massive companies.

IVF TECHNOLOGIES AND WORK PRACTICE

IVF clinics could and should be working in a streamlined and homogeneous way to ensure standardised, safe and effective treatment. This is how all routine medical practice in other specialisms takes place. Unfortunately, this is not the case in the current IVF-industry and there seems to be no indication that this will change either in the short or long-term unless some people face some hard truths. Some IVF clinics have even managed to publish fabricated or partially complete scientific data which has resulted in an increase in their market value. To go with this, there is minimal fear of prosecution (the laws probably do not exist) and there is no evidence of a duty of care to their patients. Duty of care is the bedrock of healthcare, and it states that everything a health care professional does must be in the best interests of the patient.

The only way to correct this is problem of untested and unproven 'add-ons' is for all new IVF technologies to undergo randomised controlled trials (RCT) to ensure that the new product or technology is safe and effective. This does not happen at present because such trials are expensive and may even result in a negative outcome. Instead of this cautious, professional approach, new technologies or procedures in IVF are dreamt up one day and in use on patients in IVF clinics the next. This does not happen in any other area of clinical practice and it places fertility patients in a potentially dangerous situation both medically and financially. The sad truth is that fertility patients are not only in being given untested and unproven 'treatments' but they are paying for the 'procedures' which may be totally ineffective in terms of improving the live-birth rate.

The 'Right' Patient

The choice of the 'right' patient, in terms of the right patient and the right treatment is an area which needs much more attention in IVF. Many patients embark on IVF treatment even though other options could be much more effective such as optimisation of their physical and psychological well-being. In some IVF clinics, as soon as prospective new patients walk through the door, patients are placed directly onto an IVF treatment cycle, often with many expensive 'add-ons'. Alternative treatment options are most often ignored by IVF clinics which exist for their primary purpose i.e. carrying out *in vitro* fertilisation and selling their products such as IVF, ICSI and related treatments. This is where IVF clinics create their income and profit. There is no income or profit in trying to get couples pregnant by alternative methods such as life-style changes which may involve something as simple as good advice. For example, is it truly advisable to start IVF treatment in over-weight patients, where blood sugar levels are high and who would primarily benefit from life-style changes? No, it is not! The patients should receive help and guidance to assist in weight loss when fertility very often naturally returns. The male partner may have sperm which might be of low quality because his obesity or unhealthy lifestyle. Once again, such a patient should not go directly to IVF, other options should be explored before IVF treatment. This thinking by IVF clinics needs to change to reduce unnecessary, complex, expensive treatments when they are in fact not actually needed. The snag here is that such ethical (some would even argue 'normal') medical practice would reduce the profit for the IVF clinic and this cannot be allowed for obvious reasons.

'Wobbly' Evidence

The availability of IVF on a global scale is related to the wealth of a country and the citizens in that country. This means that areas such as Sub-Saharan Africa have generally poor provision for fertility treatment despite high levels of infertility. The technology used in IVF today has changed completely from that used in 1978 making what was a long in-patient treatment now a simple out-patient procedure but still there are stagnating and overall disappointing low live birth success rates. The basic technology of IVF has nevertheless stood the test of time. Despite this, questions need to be asked about the safety and efficacy of new technologies and most importantly of 'add-ons'. Sometimes, a 'wobbly' or unreliable evidence base for new reproductive technologies is presented and deemed acceptable "because this is IVF". This philosophy is completely wrong.

There has been a recent reliable description of a possible increased risk of congenital heart defects in IVF/ICSI babies and the conclusion that birth defects are more common in IVF babies. This is not to scare people but just to provide information which is currently appearing in babies conceived using assisted conception. In addition, there are possible concerns about the effect of IVF embryo culture (which usually varies from 3 to 5 days post-fertilisation) on the genetic make-up of the human embryo. There is so much still to be learnt about IVF but most of the current IVF practitioners have little enthusiasm for this learning; they are happy to just bumble along and make lots of money from unsuspecting patients.

It is certainly possible that some IVF patients may present at the clinic with signs of depression. This is often due to the stress of discovering that they are infertile and the process they have been through up to the first visit to a fertility clinic. Patients may show signs of frustration and they do not want to talk about their experience of unsuccessful 'trial and error' treatments they may have experienced. This could be one major reason why many questionable technologies and unnecessary procedures can be sold to patients with relative ease.

A 'Re-Boot' of IVF

What about those patients with sub-optimal egg or sperm quality? Do they just get put onto an IVF treatment cycle and hope for the best? Yes. Who truly tests the various components and variables and underlying causes in such patients rigorously? No-one, or at least very few people. This is at the core of the current problems with IVF. This wider holistic approach to fertility treatment is not practised by most IVF clinics. If it was, then patients would receive a better and safer service and arguably have a better live-birth rate. They would certainly have a better overall experience of fertility treatment. A 'bumpy' body, or any other random observation, does not mean that you immediately need IVF. It means that you need more investigation, holistic treatment and if all else fails IVF.

The only approach which will correct the current problems and poor thinking in IVF is to 're-boot' the whole system starting with the patient groups for whom IVF was primarily introduced. These were patients with 'blocked tubes' as a cause of infertility, in the fertile age group of 25-32 years of age and with good sperm parameters. This approach would give a uniform starting point for testing new ideas, technology and medication and this testing would, of course, be with the informed consent of those taking part and under the guidance of the relevant ethical committees. I am not advocating random research on unsuspecting patients (this would be worse than the current stagnation we have) but if we are to make progress, the co-operation of the fertility patients currently attending IVF clinics is essential. Such an approach, with the participation of fertility patients, would provide critical data on any new idea or treatment in a group in patients where they all broadly have the same fertility problems and are all in the same age group. This is essential because we know that success in IVF is directly proportional to the female age and the diagnosis of infertility. Using such an approach, we would be able to test any new idea or treatment scientifically and approve it to be safe and effective for general patient use. This process applies in all areas of medical practice apart from IVF. Why is this? Possibly because IVF clinics 'get away' with their current practices to the detriment of patient safety and with no real information on efficacy.

The patient group which has been proposed as a 'starting point' for the re-booting of IVF (tubal infertility, aged 25-32, good sperm parameters) is known to have an IVF success rate (i.e., live-birth rate) of around 30%. If a new technology or treatment is tested on this group and it is found that the live-birth rate statistically increases above 30%, then this might be the first true advance in IVF since 1978. When things are tried in random patient groups with no baseline, then the results become blurry and over-complicated in terms of the outcome of the treatment being tested. Even the patient group with 'blocked tubes' and 'good sperm' is currently not being rigorously studied on any other potentially relevant factors they may have such as variations in ethnicities, age, Body Mass Index (BMI) smoking and alcohol intake. When this baseline is properly set, then this could then be the position from which to test each single "add on" rigorously. Using a homogenous (all with very similar diagnosis and other factors) group of patients, treated using the same stimulation protocol and subsequent treatment will allow meaningful data to be collected and safe and effective benefits handed on to future patients. This would be a true 're-boot' of IVF and would be a massive step forward for patients, but will it ever happen? In the current environment probably not, because practice has become so poor in some IVF clinics that they do not even care about their monthly pregnancy rate, patient complaint rates or live birth rates. The focus is on getting people through the door, having treatment, taking the cash and moving on to the next customer. Some patients reading this may recognise this sequence of events. It is the sign of a poor, uninspiring IVF clinic which exists only to generate profit.

TREATMENTS OF MALE INFERTILITY

Treatment for male infertility started using trial and error (no randomised controlled trial) with the introduction of Intracytoplasmic Sperm Injection (ICSI) in the early 1990's. The development of surgical sperm retrieval techniques for men with no sperm at all in their ejaculation was also developed around this time. The ICSI process requires that the sperm is selected 'by-eye' by the embryologist, who then damages the tail of the sperm to immobilise it. This is the first problem with ICSI. This sperm selection by appearance only has never been validated as being an effective way to select the 'best sperm' and at the end of the day, after a very long shift, a tired embryologist may think the best 'looking' sperm is that sperm which is easiest to catch. In IVF, the sperm selected to fertilise the egg undergoes exactly the same natural selection process as a sperm in natural conception. Having a human (sometimes a very tired human with blurry eyes) select the best sperm for fertilisation is at best a compromise and at worst, potentially damaging.

'Catching Sperm'

Another important point about catching and selecting sperm for ICSI is that sperm usually swim very quickly and without some method of 'slowing them down', it would be extremely difficult to get the chosen sperm into a needle the diameter of a human hair in as short a time as possible. The method which is used to 'slow down' sperm is to place them in fluid containing a viscous chemical called polyvinyl pyrrolidone (PVP). This is a viscous chemical which 'slows down' sperm by simply making the media more difficult to swim through. When the sperm has been caught, the embryologist will crush the tail to stop it swimming and pick it up in a tiny amount of PVP into the ICSI needle. The sperm and PVP are then directly injected into the egg using a very fine needle and expensive manipulation technology. There are two things to note here. The first is that the sperm is deliberately damaged before injection into the egg. This does not seem to have a detrimental effect on the sperm itself and it is the head of the sperm which contains the DNA needed for fertilisation. The second is that a small amount of PVP is injected directly into the egg with the sperm. PVP is also thought to be safe but in reality, no one really knows what this complex chemical does during the very early stages of human development.

It is also worth noting that the eggs which are injected with sperm using ICSI have to have the cells which naturally surround the egg (known as the cumulus cells) removed using an enzyme called hyaluronidase. It is an enzyme (a biological catalyst) which can break down the cumulus cells surrounding the egg so that the egg can be clearly seen for the sperm injection process. Once again, exposure of the egg to this enzyme could be detrimental, but it seems from a visual point of view that most eggs survive this treatment. These things are rarely, if ever, mentioned to patients who consent to ICSI. Perhaps they should be?

It is interesting that in the early days of IVF, the opinion amongst all scientists was: "don't touch the egg"! This was because that any manipulation of the egg was thought to be potentially damaging. In fact, when I worked at Bourn Hall Clinic, I was the first person to inject a human sperm beneath the transparent cover surrounding the egg called the zona pellucida. This was in an attempt to help a patient who had failed fertilisation with IVF. The sperm appeared to be attached to the zona pellucida, but they did not then penetrate the egg. When I carried out this procedure, I was under strict instructions from Bob Edwards to place the sperm underneath the zona pellucida and, in no circumstances, ever touch the egg itself. I did not crush the tail of the sperm and I did not use PVP. I followed these instructions not to touch the egg very closely and we were surprised to see that the egg fertilised and started to develop. The embryo was returned to the mother but sadly, no pregnancy resulted.

ICSI has become the standard treatment for men with low sperm counts. It has since become the standard treatment for almost everyone undergoing IVF. This is a bad thing. To include ICSI in every IVF cycle includes a considerably higher payment for the treatment and it is just possible that this might be the reason that all patients now get ICSI whether they need it or not. These patients who do not actually need ICSI, but nevertheless, are sold to them by their clinic, are also exposed to the risks associated with ICSI which I have described above.

'Add-ons'

In the following section, I will review the many and varied 'add-on' treatments to IVF, such as ICSI and also consider the more radical and perhaps unproven technology used as 'add-ons' to IVF. It is also important to consider the impact of patient pressure on the use of 'add-ons'. This is typically where a patient has a friend who got pregnant with a specific 'add-on' and that patient now insists on that 'add-on' for her own treatment. Such things are known as anecdotal reports, and the important thing to understand is that because something works for one person it does not mean it will work for someone else. Patient pressure is present in all of these 'add-ons' and some clinics even claim that they offer 'add-ons' because if they did not then patients would go elsewhere for their treatment (and the clinic would lose money). This is the total reverse of what patients should be actually thinking. A clinic which wants to throw every 'add-on' available at them as soon as they walk through the door is a clinic which should be avoided at all costs.

Intracytoplasmic Sperm Injection (ICSI) and Related Technologies

The first ICSI births were reported in 1992 as a treatment for severe male infertility. Ten years later, a follow up of babies born following ICSI indicated that ICSI seemed to be a safe procedure, although it was stated that further studies are needed to ensure long-term safety of ICSI. We will not really know if there are any implications from the use of ICSI before children born through the use of ICSI have their own children. More recently, a review of ICSI showed that there are possible higher risks of major birth defects, a possible higher risk of autism and the possibility that ICSI conceived men have lower sperm count and motility when compared to naturally conceived peers. Despite these reservations, it is clear that ICSI is the only route to treatment when there is severe male infertility (other than donor sperm) and that it may or may not have long-term risks and these will only be known in the fullness of time. The big problem in IVF is the ever-increasing use of ICSI in patients *without* severe male infertility. There is no real evidence that these patients either benefit from or may potentially be damaged by, the widespread contra-indicated use of ICSI. A Randomised Controlled Trial of ICSI *vs.* IVF in non-male factor infertility is underway to resolve these difficult questions. There is also some concern that there could be selective outcome reporting in IVF/ICSI Randomized Controlled Trials which may be resulting in false or misleading data being used in clinical practice. This has to be considered against the background of general fabrication and falsification of research data by some scientists, which unfortunately clouds the whole debate and could have a major, potentially damaging, negative impact on clinical practice. In the UK, it is reported that ICSI is used in anything from 20% to 80% of fertility treatments and in the higher percentage, there was no increased live birth rate or an increased overall fertilisation rate suggesting that the use of ICSI in these cases makes *no difference at all* to the overall outcomes.

Many clinics also recommend ICSI to all patients with low numbers of eggs (*e.g.*1-5) even when there are no male factor infertility issues. This is thought to enhance the chances of fertilisation. There is *no evidence base at all* for this practice and indeed, a recent European multicentre analysis states that the 'number of oocytes (eggs) retrieved has no value in the selection of insemination procedure in case of non-male factor infertility'.

There is, of course, a financial incentive for clinics to carry out ICSI on as many patients as possible and this could fuel the overuse or inappropriate use of ICSI by some fertility clinics. This over-use of ICSI by almost all IVF clinics on a global scale is a major scandal in IVF and something which is costing patients a vast amount of money and bringing massive profits to not only IVF clinics but also the manufacturers of the complex equipment and consumables needed to carry out ICSI.

Intracytoplasmic Morphologically Selected Sperm Injection (IMSI)

IMSI was developed in 2008, as a modification to ICSI, in an attempt to increase embryo quality and/or subsequent live birth rate in patients who had previous failed ICSI treatment cycles. It failed. IMSI is a very simple concept which just involves the selection of the sperm to be injected under a higher magnification than ICSI thus enabling the embryologist to see additional detail in the sperm head selected for injection and subsequent fertilisation of the egg. Researchers have shown in a randomized 'sibling egg' study on IMSI that IMSI does not improve fertilisation rate or embryonic development. This confirms that IMSI has no real benefit to patients despite being offered as an expensive 'add on' to routine treatment, making it even more expensive than ICSI. Further meta-analysis (this looks at all the medical publications available on a subject and brings them all together to form a coherent overall opinion on a subject) on IMSI *versus* ICSI comes to the conclusion that there is not sufficient evidence to support the use of IMSI in IVF for male infertility. This is also is supported by the most recent meta-analysis showing no difference between live birth rates and miscarriage rates in IMSI *versus* ICSI. The UK Human Fertilisation and Embryology Authority (HFEA) states that IMSI is neither effective nor safe. There are two main factors which drive the current use of IMSI despite negative literature evidence and regulatory authority opinion, these are:

- Patient pressure: These are patients with failed cycles using ICSI who seek a 'cure' to their problem and will try anything put forward by the clinic to achieve their aims. This is perhaps the most powerful driving force in this and all other 'add-ons'. If a given clinic cannot offer what the patients believe is needed, then they patients will seek it out elsewhere.
- Manufacturers of the additional equipment, consumables and training needed to provide IMSI produce a significant profit from these sales and fertility clinics in turn charge considerably more to provide IMSI.

In summary, if you are asked to pay for IMSI please do not be afraid to ask plenty of questions before you consent to this procedure. My advice to anyone is that IMSI is a pointless, expensive process which should be avoided at all costs.

Physiological Intracytoplasmic Sperm Injection (PICSI)

A second modification of ICSI, using a chemical called hyaluronan to select sperm for injection (PICSI), is offered to some patients who have had a prior failed cycle or miscarriage following ICSI. A recent parallel, two group, randomised trial has shown that PICSI does not significantly improve live birth rates and is therefore not recommended to treat fertility patients. Despite this, many clinics still offer PICSI with increased costs to the patient. The UK HFEA agree with this finding and state that PICSI is neither effective nor safe. I do not recommend PICSI to anyone.

Sperm DNA Fragmentation Testing

Many IVF clinics offer male patients sperm DNA fragmentation testing in an attempt to assess a possible cause of male infertility. This technology represents a significant income source for many IVF clinics. Despite this, the current opinion is that sperm DNA fragmentation studies *should not* be offered until randomised controlled trials prove clinical efficacy. Male patients with increased DNA fragmentation are often offered antioxidant medication in an effort to 'modify' or 'improve' their sperm DNA fragmentation. Current medical opinion states that such an approach 'may be useful' although the pregnancy rate in such patients is low. There is currently conflicting evidence on the value of sperm DNA fragmentation testing and the results of this 'add-on' are not thought to be important in the treatment plan of fertility patients. In summary, sperm DNA fragmentation testing is an expensive 'add-on' which will make no difference whatsoever to your live birth outcome. I do not recommend sperm DNA fragmentation tests to anyone.

Time-Lapse Video Analysis of Embryonic Development

This is arguably the most ridiculous and expensive 'add-on' in the current practice of IVF. Time-lapse video analysis and un-interrupted culture of developing human embryos is now routine in most IVF clinics and patient pressure to use the technology is extremely high. There is, however, still great controversy as to how much time-lapse and un-interrupted embryo culture actually produces better results in relation to the many other parameters involved in embryo culture. The HFEA state that at present, there is not enough evidence that time-lapse video analysis has any overall impact on live-birth rates and therefore the additional cost of the process is not worthwhile. Despite this, most patients want to use time-lapse technology in their treatment and may even change clinics if their current clinic cannot provide time-lapse technology. Further development in time-lapse recording and image analysis in the future may provide a benefit to patients, but at present, such technology is unavailable. In summary, time-lapse monitoring of your embryos during development is a pointless process which will not increase your live birth rate at all. Please avoid it.

Pre-Implantation Genetic Screening (PGS) and Preimplantation Genetic Diagnosis (PGD)

Pre-Implantation Genetic Screening (Aneuploidy Screening)

PGS was first described in 1996 as a possible way to identify embryos which have incorrect number of chromosomes. PGS was then known as aneuploidy screening which is a scientific term referring to abnormal chromosome numbers. It was initially proposed for older female patients and therefore possibly increased the live birth rate in this patient group. It did not. There is of course a significant cost implication to patients who decide to use PGS. This is because the embryo has to undergo biopsy and the resultant biopsy is then analysed by another highly specialised laboratory. More recent analysis of the data obtained from PGS and the resulting possible benefits to patients concludes that the overall use of PGS in the clinical practice of IVF is increasingly difficult to justify.

The HFEA state that there is conflicting evidence on the safety and efficacy of PGS. Most worrying is a recent report that 'abnormal' PGS embryos can actually go on to produce normal, healthy live-births and that PGS, therefore, results in the disposal of many normal embryos. My advice is to avoid PGS or aneuploidy screening; it has no clear benefit to any patients.

Pre-Implantation Genetic Diagnosis (PGD)

PGD is the diagnosis of disease in embryos with a view to excluding serious genetically inherited disease. This is a very different story. So much so that it arguably should not be in a critical discussion of IVF 'add-ons' but I add it here because it is a very important technology for people who carry genetic diseases. The basic technology is the same as PGS, but the analysis is very different and looks for genes carrying disease and not just a simple assessment of chromosome number. In theory, it is possible to screen for any genetic disease where the genes are known and as of today, at least 600 different genetic diseases can be screened for using PGD. This enables families with known genetic diseases to have healthy children. It is also possible to offer Pre-implantation Tissue Testing (PTT) in families where a 'saviour sibling' is needed to provide umbilical cord blood for transplantation to treat blood disorders. PGD and PTT are examples of excellent, safe and effective treatments which have saved and transformed many lives. The technology is advanced and relatively expensive, but the benefits to patients are enormous and the safety and efficacy are completely proven. If anyone finds themselves in need of such technology, then there are several centres of excellence around the world offering the service. It is safe, effective and certainly **not** a pointless 'add-on'.

Endometrial 'scratching' (Endometrial Injury)

Endometrial 'scratching' was first introduced in 2003 as a proposed way of enhancing the receptivity of the endometrium to the implanting embryo. It has since been shown to have no beneficial effect and has no biological basis. Despite this, the 'scratch' is still widely offered in fertility clinics, often with a disproportionate fee attached to it, and patients are trusting clinics that this might help in their treatment. The HFEA state that there is conflicting evidence regarding endometrial scratching and further research is needed. I do not recommend the 'scratch' to anyone. It is a pointless process.

Assisted Hatching

Assisted hatching is the cutting or opening of the transparent 'shell' (called the zona pellucida) around an embryo using acid, laser or other tools. The proposed purpose of assisted hatching is that it may help hatching; this is the process which the embryo must undergo to enhance implantation into the womb. More recently, a meta-analysis of laser assisted hatching came to the conclusion that large scale, prospective, randomized controlled trials are needed to determine if assisted hatching is clinically relevant. The HFEA states that there is no evidence that assisted hatching is either effective or safe and the National Institute for Clinical Excellence (NICE) states: "Assisted hatching is not recommended because it has not been shown to improve pregnancy rates." Despite these opinions, and the highly conflicting medical literature, many clinics still promote assisted hatching to their patients as a possible treatment modality and charge an 'add-on' fee for the service. I do not recommend assisted hatching to anyone under any circumstances.

Embryo Glue

'Embryo glue' is a modified embryo culture medium used at the time of embryo transfer, which is proposed to enhance the process of implantation in the womb. The medical literature is conflicting on the use of embryo glue and the HFEA states that further research is required to confirm safety and efficacy. Embryo glue is often offered to patients who have had a previous failed IVF cycle despite the evidence that it will not help such patients. I do not recommend embryo glue to anyone. It is untested and unproven.

Elective Freeze All Cycles

Elective freeze all cycles involve the creation of a batch of fresh embryos for a patient and then freezing all of these embryos for the future frozen embryo transfer at a later date. Such an approach may be useful in those patients at risk of the ovarian hyper-stimulation syndrome (OHSS) but not for those patients who are either normal or poor responders to ovarian stimulation. The HFEA state that there is conflicting evidence for elective freeze-all cycles and further research is needed. If this 'add on' is offered to patients who do not need it, then it will incur further costs on their treatment and the risk of embryo damage during the freezing and thawing process. Unless clinically indicated (and this will be rare), I do not recommend elective freezing cycles to anyone.

Reproductive Immunology

Some IVF practitioners believe that manipulation of the female patients' immune system may result in an increase in fertility by reducing the activity of cells known to immunologists as Natural Killer (NK) cells. The evidence in support of this concept is conflicting and many consider that reproductive immunology intervention should only be part of clinical research. This is a sensible approach. Such interventions in immunology include the administration of the steroid prednisolone, intravenous immunoglobulin (IVIg), Tumour Necrosis Factor Alpha (TNFα) antagonists, partner lymphocyte immunisation and Intralipid infusions. Most recently a systematic review of immune therapies in the treatment of infertility raises the point of a need for better immunological diagnosis and the follow-up of infants born following immunological interventions. It is also worth noting that the physician you will see in a fertility clinic is almost always trained in obstetrics and gynaecology. This is fine if your treatment is IVF. However, he or she has very little training in clinical immunology and as such, should not be making immunological decisions on your behalf. This is like consulting an orthopaedic surgeon for a heart transplant, not a good idea. Some of the gynaecologists in fertility clinics will claim that they fully understand clinical immunology and their ego will happily agree with them. Their peers would not agree with them, and neither do the regulatory authorities. If you are to receive immunological treatment (which is almost certainly a waste of time and money in fertility treatment) then you should be supervised by a fully qualified Clinical Immunologist. This is for your own safety. The HFEA state that there is no evidence that reproductive immunology interventions are either safe or effective and all of the interventions carry risk. The cost of these reproductive immunology interventions is high and represents a significant income source in some IVF clinics. I do not recommend any immunological 'treatments' to anyone until a clear demonstration of a clear benefit has been shown in the future.

Acupuncture

The proposition that acupuncture might assist in the treatment of fertility patients has resulted in the use of the technology for many years despite any clear rationale or benefit of use. Acupuncture may have side benefits such as promoting relaxation, stress reduction and general well-being, but it should not be used if the context is to enhance live birth rates, or improve sperm counts or treat anything in infertility.

CONCLUSIONS ON 'ADD-ONS'

Basic IVF, as developed by Edwards, Steptoe and Purdy, is clearly a safe procedure (we now have over 40 years of data), providing the option of a family to millions of people around the world which would not otherwise be possible. The only thing we still need to see is the reproductive abilities of people conceived by IVF but at present, this seems to be comparable with the rest of the population. There are many drivers to the use of the 'add-ons' described above in IVF, including clinics who wish to optimise their income, manufacturers who only see profits and do not worry about patients and most surprisingly of all the patients themselves. Fertility patients are very vulnerable and will do anything to meet their desire for a family. They put their trust in fertility clinics, and if a clinic recommends an 'add-on', regardless of cost, safety or efficacy, then the patients will accept the advice and pay for the 'add-on'. Fertility patients also see and contribute to online discussions which are totally unregulated, and opinions and advice from this source drive them to ask for 'add-ons' to 'increase' their chances of success. This is a unique and unacceptable type of medical practice similar to some dentists in the past who may offer inappropriate treatment simply for profit. It is also more convenient for IVF specialists to directly implement questionable IVF technologies and blame such things as natural killer cells for an implantation failure which needs an expensive and untested 'remedy'. This is instead of telling patients that life-style interventions might better optimise their egg, sperm, womb lining and overall body health. This may lead to improved fertility treatment outcome without the need for expensive, unproven and possibly harmful interventions. This is especially in those patients with the diagnosis of sub-fertility or unexplained (idiopathic) infertility.

The clarity of information available to fertility patients in some clinics is also a serious concern in the context of 'add-ons'. Regulatory authorities such as the HFEA have very clear advice on 'add-ons' to patients, but despite this, patients still request 'add-ons' which are untested for efficacy and safety, and clinics encourage these requests and ensure that they have all of the 'add-ons' available. A good example is time lapse monitoring of embryonic development which almost all patients request because they are convinced that it will help their treatment. Many fertility clinics sadly offer time-lapse to every patient as if it is tried and tested technology, it is not. Those clinics without time lapse equipment, or those who choose not to offer it because they understand that it is a pointless 'add-on', often lose patients to other clinics who do offer time lapse. This simple example results in patients paying for an unnecessary procedure and even changing clinics to get the 'add-on'. Manufacturers are selling their equipment to clinics with enormous profits. This cycle of patient demand and manufacturer greed supports the continued use of pointless, ineffective 'add-ons'.

MISLEADING

The problem in IVF clinics is that fertility patients are being seriously (and possibly deliberately and unlawfully) misled and the clinics and manufacturers benefit from this poor behaviour and clinical malpractice.

Regulators, such as the HFEA in the UK, have clear opinions and information on the safety and efficacy IVF 'add-ons', but they do not enforce these restrictions in clinics. They sometimes express reservations and concerns with individual clinics during and after licensing inspections but they do not enforce these opinions with the backing of the law. It is important that regulators must be more pro-active to protect patients from untested and unproven 'add-ons' and to provide the protection that fertility patients need and deserve. Regulators must send a very clear message to clinics who are generating significant income by promoting untested and unproven 'add-ons' that their practice is unacceptable.

Many fertility practitioners will point to 'evidence' which shows that their 'add-ons' are safe and effective. The patients are unable to critically appraise such information and in some cases the evidence might even be biased or, worse still, fake. Fake, manipulated or totally fabricated scientific data seems to be becoming an increasing trend and fertility practitioners must bear this in mind when making clinical decisions and advising patients.

The only 'add-on' in the discussion above which should be used in routine clinical practice is pre-implantation genetic diagnosis (PGD). This procedure is offered to patients who carry genes for specific diseases and very often, they have no fertility problems. It is therefore arguable that PGD is not a fertility treatment and, as such, should not be part of the current debate on IVF 'add-ons' as described above. The rest of the 'add-ons' described, *including ICSI with no clinical indication*, are ineffective and unsafe and should not be used in clinical practice.

COUNSELLING AND CLINICAL TRIALS

The level of counselling in IVF is poor because, unless counselling is mandatory, most fertility patients do not take advantage of counselling. I propose that all patients considering 'add-ons' should undergo mandatory counselling to ensure that they receive unbiased advice on the safety and efficacy of the 'add-on' being considered. I have mentioned many times before that IVF clinic counsellors are sadly underused and this is another great example where they could have a considerable beneficial effect on fertility patients.

Some IVF practitioners propose that 'multi-centre' clinical trials must be carried out in order to properly assess IVF 'add-ons'. The inherent problem with this clinical trial approach in IVF is that clinics all use different stimulation protocols, they have different timing of ovulation induction and they are situated in different climate regions and elevations (air pressure could impact culture media as do different room temperatures or air particles). They are also staffed by a wide range of people with varying skills and abilities. They all use different culture media and the timing of such things as fertilization with IVF or ICSI differ. This is the so called 'heterogeneous' or mixed population of patients and technologies, which means that drawing any clear conclusions from the resulting data is virtually impossible. Only a homogeneous population as described earlier will result in interesting and informative data.

If such studies are to be carried out, then there must be a standardisation of conditions in fertility clinical trials so that the data collected will be comparable and relevant. It is essential to include sufficient patient numbers in every single study to get the statistical power needed to make firm conclusions.

STARTING FROM SCRATCH AND 'BLOBS'

Starting from scratch, or a 're-boot' of IVF might be wishful thinking and not manageable at all. Take the example of IMSI. This proposes to predict embryo quality depending on the size and numbers of small 'blobs' (known technically as vacuoles) seen in sperm. It was found that those sperm with certain types and numbers of 'blobs' influenced embryo development to the blastocyst stage. These findings raised many questions: Will it be possible to prospectively and deliberately inject sperm with various 'blobs' into oocytes? No. Who would dare or risk to do so? No-one. Which ethical committee would give the green light for such a study on a large scale? None. This kind of experimentation on human eggs and sperm is unethical and illegal in most countries. This stance protects patients, and I completely agree with this position, but at the same time, it means that we will never know if procedures such as IMSI have any benefit or not.

This is one of many examples from the world of IVF, and it is provided as a thought-provoking concept. The purpose is to explain some of the difficulties faced in modern IVF. It may also stimulate new discussions on what is practical to achieve in the future of IVF and what we have to accept as 'given' based on current knowledge and medical publications available in IVF.

The conclusion has to be that the current and growing number of 'add-ons' in IVF is unacceptable and poses a significant risk to the medical and financial safety of patients. It is driven by patient pressure, corporate greed and the need for clinics to optimise their income. It is critical that regulatory authorities intervene in this 'vicious circle' to protect patients and that going forward any new 'add-on' must be supported by clear evidence of safety and efficacy *before* it is introduced. This might be impossible or very hard to accomplish, but the safety of fertility patients is the prime objective.

KEY POINTS OF CHAPTER 7

- Add-ons are untested and unproven, but they are in routine use in almost all fertility clinics at a great financial cost to patients.
- There are many different 'add-ons' and new ones are being developed all the time.
- Patients need to be aware of the 'add-on' problem and to ask the right questions at the right time to avoid being dragged into the shady world of 'add-ons'.
- Fertility patients should take advice from as many healthcare professionals as possible about 'add-ons', including the impartial fertility clinic counsellor.

CHAPTER 8

The Regulators and Professional Societies

Peter Hollands

(The Role of Regulators and Professional Societies in the Treatment of Infertility)

Law is order, and good law is good order.
Aristotle

Summary: This chapter explores the importance of regulation and professional societies in the safe and effective delivery of IVF. An overview of the key activities of regulatory authorities is discussed to illustrate their importance in fertility treatment.

INTRODUCTION

When IVF was first used in 1978 to create the first IVF baby, this was the result of exceptional scientific and medical expertise. Bob Edwards and Jean Purdy brought their considerable and unique scientific skills developed over decades of research and development and Patrick Steptoe brought his surgical skill and technology, without which it would have been impossible to get access to human eggs. This was, of course, laparoscopy, which has since been replaced by ultrasound guided egg collection. Despite this, the principle of laparoscopy continues to be used in other applications in surgical practice today. This combination of experience and technology resulted in a completely new medical procedure which operated at the very epicentre of human life: The process of human reproduction *in vitro*.

POWER IS NOT ALWAYS A GOOD THING

The introduction of IVF meant that scientists and physicians now had the power to manipulate human reproduction. As such, they had considerable power for good to help infertile patients. There was also the potential power for undesirable activities such as the possibility of human cloning, using animals to carry human embryos and many other highly undesirable possibilities which can arise from IVF technology. It was clear from the very start that IVF needs independent, external regulators to ensure both patient safety and quality of treatment and that no undesirable or dangerous technology was applied to human reproduction.

When Bourn Hall Clinic began operations in the early 1980's, it was the first ever IVF clinic in the world, and it began to operate without any regulation at all. We are all certainly very fortunate that Bob Edwards, Jean Purdy and Patrick Steptoe were meticulous in their requirement that everything which was done must be as safe as possible (based on the limited knowledge at that time) and nothing must be done which may interfere with the otherwise natural process of human reproduction. The people who first called for regulation of IVF were Edwards, Steptoe and Purdy because they knew that the technology could easily be abused and in the wrong hands may threaten the very basis and safety of human reproduction.

UK REGULATION

The first step in the regulation of IVF in the UK came in the form of a Voluntary Regulatory Authority (VLA) following the report of the Warnock Report in 1984. The Voluntary or Interim Licensing Authority was introduced in 1985. Bourn Hall Clinic supported and welcomed this innovation as a welcome step towards formal mandatory licensing and worked very closely with the VLA. In the UK, there then followed new laws relating to assisted conception which were passed in 1991 and the creation of the Human Embryology and Fertilisation Authority (HFEA) in 1991. The HFEA is a respected and competent regulatory authority in the UK, and it was the gold-standard basis of similar regulatory authorities in other countries which now regulate IVF on a global scale. Today, the IVF industry is regulated in most countries, and the main role is to protect the safety of patients and to ensure that the quality and effectiveness of treatments are always at the absolute optimum. Regulatory authorities also monitor the creation and rate of multiple pregnancies by IVF clinics because such multiple pregnancies have significant risks for both the mother and babies. Most IVF patients now receive just one embryo at embryo transfer, with two or more embryos only allowed in specific circumstances.

THE ROLE OF A REGULATORY AUTHORITY

It is useful to briefly describe the many and varied things which a regulatory authority does in order to fully understand the importance of regulatory authorities in IVF treatment and how they are a fantastic resource for all fertility patients.

In your fertility clinic, you should be able to see the Regulatory License (*e.g.*, in the UK this will be the HFEA) displayed very clearly, usually somewhere such as the general reception area. Most clinics are inspected when they first open and thereafter re-inspected every 2-3 years or sooner if a specific problem arises, which is of concern to the regulatory authority. The date of the inspection and the date of the next planned inspection should be clear on the license. The license should list the procedures for which a clinic is licensed (not every clinic is licensed for every possible procedure in IVF) and it will also state who the Person Responsible is. The Person Responsible is usually a senior physician or scientist and this person has the legal responsibility for the safe and proper treatment of patients under the license. In the UK, and most other countries, the license is linked to relevant laws and if the clinic contravenes those laws, then the Person Responsible could be charged with a criminal offence. This reflects the importance of regulation and the power behind it. Regulation has developed in this way with the prime objective to protect fertility patients and to ensure that the treatment offered is safe and effective. This becomes a bit of a grey area when considering the use of 'add-ons' discussed in Chapter 7, but for the rest of the routine fertility treatment, the law is strictly applied. It is my sincere hope that the regulatory will clamp down hard on 'add-ons' very soon.

What Does the Regulatory Authority Regulate?

The regulatory authorities, such as the HFEA in the UK, regulate every aspect of fertility treatment, but it is worth spending a few moments to properly understand what this actually means. The HFEA, for example, publishes a Code of Practice which covers everything which is inspected in the clinic, and these items relate to relevant laws. It is beyond the scope of this book to discuss the Code of Practice in detail (and every other regulatory authority will have a similar document to the Code of Practice) but it is interesting to mention a few.

The regulations describe how many staff are needed in an IVF clinic (depending on the workload of the clinic) and their qualifications, experience and competence. This competence must be regularly assessed. This ensures that when you speak to any of the staff in the fertility clinic, you can be reassured that you are speaking to someone who is qualified and competent in their area of expertise.

The counselling available at the clinic and other areas of patient support are described in the Code of Practice, but as described earlier, the clinic counsellors are sadly underused because even though the clinic is duty bound to offer counselling the fertility patients do not have to accept the offer. I would like to see this change to a situation where fertility patients all accept the offer of counselling because I believe that all patients would benefit immensely.

Consent is a critical area of fertility treatment and all fertility patients should be familiar with the consent forms, and should understand the consent they have given for their treatment. Such consent ranges from consent for the treatment itself all the way to the area such as disclosure of information to third parties. You will be taken through the consent process by a fertility nurse and if you have questions, please do not hesitate to ask as consent is extremely important.

The regulatory authority also defines the legal parenthood of any babies born as a result of IVF. This may be very straight forward if the patients are married and not using donor gametes, but it can be very complex, especially when donor gametes or surrogates are involved. This again is an area which will be discussed with you face to face with an experienced fertility nurse because when your baby is born, you must be sure that you are the legal parents. This may sound a bit scary, but it is not. Your clinic will take you through the forms and the process, but once again, it is an area which asks for concentration and understanding and as always, if you have any questions, then do ask.

In the past few years, the regulatory authorities have become very involved in the minimisation of multiple births following IVF. When I first practised IVF in Bourn Hall Clinic, we would often replace three, sometimes even four embryos because back then it was thought that more embryos meant a better success rate. More recently the regulatory authorities have stopped this practice because it does not increase overall success rates and it places the mother at increased risk of multiple pregnancy. Multiple pregnancy has medical risks for the mother and baby, and it also has financial implications because neo-natal intensive care is an extremely expensive service to provide. As a result, most IVF clinics today replace just one embryo, sometimes two if the patient is older or has other past history and extremely rarely three embryos. The balance is between making sure of the safety of the mother and baby and optimising IVF success rates. The increased use of blastocyst replacement in IVF clinics means that the best 'looking' embryo can easily be selected, thus optimising the chance of establishing a pregnancy. It is worth mentioning that even if one embryo is replaced there is still the possibility of identical twins; this is rare but certainly not impossible.

An important area covered by the regulatory authorities is that of welfare of the child. This may sound a bit strange because fertility patients are totally focussed on a family and would certainly give complete love and affection to any baby they produce using fertility treatment. Despite this, there are may be circumstances where one or another patient has a past history which might suggest that they might struggle with being a parent or need additional support should they become a parent. This is not something to worry about and if there are any issues, then your fertility clinic will support you through the process and ensure that everyone is satisfied with the welfare of the child requirements.

Embryo testing and sex selection are monitored very closely by the regulatory authorities. In terms of embryo testing, they require a considerable information to be provided by clinics about how many embryos are being tested, what they are being tested for and the training and competence of the embryologist carrying out the testing. This ensures that everything is fully documented and that everything is carried out to the utmost levels of safety and quality. Sex selection of embryos, for the purpose of selecting the sex of the baby for social reasons, is illegal in most countries and the UK led the way in this prohibition. The reason for this is that if fertility clinics only replaced embryos of a certain sex, then eventually, this would imbalance the male to female ratio of the human race. The only situation where sex selection may be used is in patients who carry known genetic diseases such as haemophilia where the male babies suffer from the disease. By not replacing male embryos in these patients, it should be possible to avoid haemophilia. As modern diagnostics advance, it will be possible to identify the haemophilia gene in developing embryos, so even in this context sex selection will not need to be used.

Many fertility treatments available today use donor gametes (eggs and sperm) and the regulatory oversee this process. Donors must be properly recruited, they must have medical examinations and detailed blood tests to exclude any possible diseases being passed on, and they must be very clear about the implications of being a gamete donor. In this way, the regulatory authority protects the safety of both donors and recipient patients.

Surrogacy is often needed by fertility patients, especially in those female patients who have previously undergone a hysterectomy or some same sex patients. The process of surrogacy is complex from a legal, financial and emotional point of view and the regulatory authorities help to ensure that the surrogate, the parents and the resulting baby are all safe. If you need to use surrogacy then your clinic staff will carefully guide you through the process and ensure that all legal regulatory requirements are met.

The basic activities of an IVF clinic involve obtaining gametes (eggs and sperm), processing the gametes, sometimes storing them and sometimes transporting them. These may sound like simple procedures, but in actual fact, they require a lot of expertise from physicians, embryologists and nurses and the related documentation and record keeping is very complex. The regulatory authorities monitor these activities very closely to ensure that your gametes are handled skilfully and safely.

The process of IVF requires high levels of traceability. This means that it must be possible to follow the process, for each pair of patients, with absolute confidence from the point of egg collection and sperm production to the point of embryo transfer, embryo freezing and if needed embryo thawing and frozen embryo replacement. Most of these records are now electronic making them very reliable and safe but once again, the regulatory authority ensures that the traceability with the fertility clinic is at the highest level. An important part of traceability is the witnessing process. Patients will be familiar with this; for example, when the female goes to egg collections, there are detailed witnessed identity checks, and a similar thing happens when the male is taken to the men's room for sperm production. Witnessing continues in detail throughout every laboratory procedure, usually using electronic systems, to ensure that there are no 'mix-ups' in the lab. Looking back, I am sure that there must have been errors in witnessing and traceability in the past but the purpose of the current regulations and the ever improving electronic witnessing systems is to ensure that today the level of witnessing and traceability are at the highest levels of reliability.

The subject of ICSI is of special interest to the regulatory authorities because it introduces increased levels of complexity above basic IVF. The main difference is the ICSI process itself which is technically more difficult than IVF and requires specifically trained and competent embryologists. There is also regulation on the mixing of IVF and ICSI embryos at embryo replacement so that the data collected on IVF and ICSI births are not confused. The clinics all have to report their ICSI data to the regulatory authorities so that an independent review of the treatment can be maintained.

Every IVF clinic must operate using something known as a Quality Management System (QMS). This is most commonly now an electronic system but at the start, it was a paper-based system. The QMS consists of all of the documents, forms, records, instructions (called Standard Operating Procedures), and analysis of the data. This ensures that the operating systems of the clinic are at the absolute optimal levels of safety and reliability and that everyone in the clinic can refer to controlled documentation when needed.

The actual premises in which the fertility clinic is carefully assessed by the regulatory authorities to ensure that they are safe and appropriate for fertility patients. There are some very specific requirements such as the build and quality of the laboratory and operating theatre and other considerations such as the general infection control within the clinic. Most fertility clinics try to make their clinic as appealing as possible to their patients, Bourn Hall Clinic is certainly a beautiful place to be, but it is reassuring that the regulatory authorities not only think about aesthetic concerns but also the extremely important technical aspects of the clinic.

This is just a very brief overview of the activity of a fertility clinic regulatory authority, but it gives a general idea of the scope and importance of their work. If you need to know more about regulatory aspects, then either ask at your clinic or contact the regulatory authority directly who are always very happy to hear from patients and have considerable resources and expertise to offer.

The European Society for Human Reproduction and Embryology (ESHRE)

ESHRE was created in 1984 by Bob Edwards and his colleagues across Europe. The purpose of the society was to allow annual conferences and discussions with everyone in Europe working in IVF. The first international meeting of ESHRE was in Bonn, Germany, in 1985 and there were approximately 50-60 delegates. I attended this first meeting and presented some data on stem cells from my Ph.D. at Cambridge University. Today the ESHRE conferences attract thousands of delegates and are held annually in various cities around Europe with a massive associated trade show. It is a very big business. In 2020 and 2021, the ESHRE conference was held virtually because of the restrictions surrounding COVID-19. ESHRE also provides training for clinical embryologists, which is recognised internationally and is an important route to qualification for some embryologists. ESHRE encouraged the formation of many similar organisations such as The American Society for Reproductive Medicine (ASRM) which provides information both for healthcare professionals and for patients. These societies are important globally so that people working in IVF can interact and share their experiences which in turn increases the quality and safety of the service offered to fertility patients.

KEY POINTS OF CHAPTER 8

- Regulation is very important in the delivery of IVF because it provides the ultimate protection to fertility patients.
- Regulation prevents the exploits of 'maverick' scientists.
- Professional societies provide an important forum where people working in infertility can obtain training, discuss new concepts and share experiences.

CHAPTER 9

The Patient 'Journey'

Peter Hollands

(What to Expect in an IVF Treatment Cycle)

Life is a journey that have a lot different paths, but any path you choose use it as your destiny.
Ryan Leonard

Summary: This chapter describes the ups and downs of a 'typical' IVF treatment cycle, but it must be noted that there may be many variations between what is described below and what was described earlier in an actual treatment cycle. This is because wherever possible, the best IVF clinics treat patients as individuals. This means that the treatment is ideally customised for the patient and is not a generic recipe which is simply repeated on everyone

THE JOURNEY

People often talk about their 'journey' as a description of what they had to go through to achieve a particular goal in life. Such expressions are rampant in reality TV for anything from baking to making pots or becoming the next pop 'sensation' or the best amateur dancer. Everyone seems to have a journey to go on! Despite this, to use this kind of terminology in the context of what is a highly stressful and technical procedure may be inappropriate. Nevertheless, if it helps fertility patients and makes the process a little easier to rationalise, then I have no objection to it. It might be better to consider fertility treatment for what it is, which is a highly technical medical procedure in the same category as minor surgery. Fertility treatment should not threaten your health (unless you are very unlucky and suffer severe OHSS), but at the same time, it is invasive and therefore does carry some risks. As a society, we have become extremely risk averse and expect the things we do not to carry risk. This is an incorrect philosophy. Everything carries some level of risk and fertility treatment is no exception. Patients must accept this as their first step to retaining their sanity during fertility treatment.

In everything I do as a healthcare professional, I place the patient at the centre, and the welfare and safety of the patient are paramount. Anything which is done, is done for the benefit of the patient. It is not done for the benefit of myself, the clinic, the owners of the clinic or anyone else; it is done for the patient. This is the duty of care which all healthcare professionals have for their patients. This is the philosophy I learnt from Edwards, Purdy and Steptoe and it is fundamental to safe, ethical and compassionate healthcare. If you feel that your clinic or your healthcare providers are not giving you their duty of care, then do not be afraid the challenge them and if you are unhappy with their reply then walk away. There are plenty more clinics and healthcare professionals out there who put duty of care at the very top of their priorities.

Many patients come into IVF treatment with little prior knowledge of the process apart from what they may have heard from other patients, family or friends. There are, of course, many books about the subject (some are better than others!) and the internet and social media contain a considerable amount of information. The problem is that much of the internet information is unreliable and social media only adds to the confusion with considerable amounts of 'fake news'. Anecdotal reports such as 'this worked for me' or 'try this clinic; I got pregnant at the first attempt' are totally unhelpful and are best ignored. I would ask all fertility patients to be very selective and critical about any information they come across, especially if it is internet based. The information coming out of fertility clinics should be broadly reliable (apart from some of that relating to some 'add-ons'), but once again, do not assume that clinic information is perfect, be critical and ask questions. The 'journey' will not be smooth; it will be tough with many ups and downs and developing this level of understanding and mind-set before you begin treatment will help you immensely in coping with the process. Be positive but do not expect everything to be perfect; in the fertility business that is a recipe for disaster.

First Things First

Everyone assumes that they are fertile and that when the time is right, they will exercise this fertility to produce children on demand. No problems are envisaged and in around 80% of people, there are no problems. A pregnancy results and not much more is thought about the process of conception. Nevertheless, many people find that despite many efforts to become pregnant over 2-3 years, they are unable to get pregnant and this is the first step in the fertility journey. The accepted general definition of infertility is the inability to develop a pregnancy after at least 1 year of trying to conceive. Some people suggest that 2 years of trying to conceive is a better marker of infertility. What is important here is that people should not be arriving at an IVF clinic when they have tried to get pregnant for 2-

3 months and are in the early 20's but have failed to establish a pregnancy. Such people should be turned away by an ethical IVF clinic and asked to return in 1 year when further investigations can begin if a pregnancy has not occurred in the meantime. Sadly, not all IVF clinics operate in this way and simply see new patients as the opportunity to generate easy profit. Before the patients know it, they are starting their first, totally inappropriate and mis-timed, IVF treatment cycle. If you find yourself hurried or rushed into IVF treatment, then please walk away and consult another clinic. There are more people out there who will treat you properly and appropriately.

Time is Running Out!

The problem with fertility treatment (and this specifically applies to the female patient) is that as the female gets older, the chance of establishing a natural pregnancy decreases considerably. There is also an additional worry in that as the female gets older, especially 40 and above, the risk of complications in pregnancy and delivery increases, as does the risk of developing Down's syndrome in the baby. Modern lifestyles also often result in couples who do not even consider starting a family until their mid-to-late 30's. The result of all of this is that most patients, by the time they find themselves at an IVF clinic, are in their mid-to-late 30's and the perceived urgency for treatment, especially for the female, is extremely high. This is a very real situation for many fertility patients and represents a considerable source of stress. In this situation, it may be necessary and sensible to proceed to IVF more quickly than would be otherwise desirable and this is left to the clinical decision of the physician who sees the patient. This may be a lesson to us all in that the reproductive window for female humans is relatively short compared to the total lifespan. A human female is fertile and legally able to have a child from 16 in the UK and by about the age of 38 it is either very difficult or impossible to become pregnant. This gives about 22 years of potential fertility, which is 27% of the current expected lifespan of a woman in the UK of 82 years. Most women do not wish to be pregnant before their early 20's or later, thus reducing this period of fertility even further. The window of fertility is very narrow, and in this time period, she has to find a partner, develop a career and keep healthy. We should perhaps think more about this in our overall understanding of reproduction and the modern lifestyle and the pressures it puts on the human female.

The First Consultation

The first step in the journey is the first consultation. This will be with a senior member of the medical team who will need to ask both partners questions about every aspect of their health, past and present, and to examine each partner. There will then be several investigations which will include blood tests for both partners (including blood tests for infectious diseases which are required by the regulatory authority), scans for the female partner and for the male partner's semen analysis. This semen analysis is often the first of such investigations for the male partner. It may seem a little strange to be asked to masturbate and ejaculate into a plastic pot, but rest assured, this is routine in an IVF clinic and not a matter of either worry or embarrassment. All of this information is then collated so that the physician can come to an initial diagnosis.

The Second and Nurse Consultation

At the second consultation with a physician, it should be possible to provide a diagnosis of the cause of infertility and an initial treatment plan. In terms of the cause of infertility, this can basically be either male factor, female factor or both. If the diagnosis is male factor, then the underlying cause will be one of those mentioned in Chapter 3 and if it is a female factor, then one of those causes mentioned in Chapter 2. There is one other category called idiopathic infertility. Idiopathic is a term used across the whole of medicine where the cause of the problem is unknown. Whatever the diagnosis, you will be provided at this point with a personalised treatment plan. It is at this stage that you will also need to complete many official forms from the regulator (the HFEA in the UK). These regulatory and consent forms are complex, and a fertility nurse is always on hand to assist in their proper completion. These forms are extremely important and any mistakes at this stage could impact your treatment and legal rights during and following treatment. The next step is then to have what is known as a 'nurse consultation'. In the nurse consultation, you will get much more detail and it is often very much more relaxed than the formal physician consultation. You will be given detailed information about your own particular treatment cycle along with instructions about your medication. In modern IVF practice, all patients administer their own prescribed medication and this is mainly to be given to the female partner. The medication is mainly injected so the female partner or her partner needs to learn how to do this. Some medications are in pessary form (inserted into the vagina) and some may be 'sniffed' into the nose. Some medication has to be administered at very specific times of day and if this timing is not adhered to, then this can have a negative effect on the outcome. Whatever the medication and the route of administration, this is an absolutely critical part of IVF treatment which needs full concentration and understanding by the patients. You will either be provided with written instructions on when to take medication or some clinics now have apps which remind patients about medication through their mobile phone.

At Last! The Treatment is Starting!

The next step when all of these preliminary things have been discussed, forms filled, payments made, and new skills acquired is to start the treatment cycle itself. The treatment cycle begins with the start of the start of the menstrual cycle and from the point of view of the treatment, the day on which menstruation starts is called Day 0. At this point, the female patient will have to begin self-medication (usually be injection) which in itself could be very stressful. If you are worried about self-medication, please talk to your fertility clinic staff, they should be very happy to help and give advice. The clinic staff are able to support you on any aspect of your treatment. There will also be many journeys to and from the clinic for scan appointments and some possible additional blood tests along the way.

The Day of Egg Collection

This is possibly one of the most stressful times in an IVF treatment cycle. On this day the female patient faces a surgical procedure, and this may be the first time she will experience such a procedure, and the male patient has to produce a semen sample on demand. At this point in the 'journey', it is extremely important that you have total trust and faith in the staff at the IVF clinic who will be caring for you. This might sound obvious, but many patients feel extremely vulnerable at this stage. If you are worried, stressed or cannot cope with anything then speak to the clinic staff. You will hopefully receive support, understanding and re-assurance from confident, skilled professional staff. Another thing which many people worry about on the day of egg collection is how many eggs will be collected? The basic rule here is that the important thing is quality and not quantity. I have seen patients producing over 40 eggs at egg collection, but this is generally a bad thing. It increases your risk of developing OHSS and many of those eggs are likely to be immature and therefore incapable of being fertilised. I think that a perfect number of eggs is around 5-10. This is because I and many others have found that these numbers produce the best eggs and the best overall outcomes. There is even a trend towards 'natural' IVF where the patients either receive extremely low, or no medication and they will therefore produce perhaps 1-2 eggs maximum. The concept here is that producing eggs naturally may produce better quality eggs. I like the idea of 'natural' IVF, but it is not suitable for everyone and it is best to discuss it with your clinic if you would like to be considered for 'natural' IVF.

Following the egg collection, the female patient will spend a short time in recovery being closely monitored and once she is stable then both male and female patients can go home. The work now starts in the lab! This will involve mixing the egg and sperm together for IVF or injection of a single sperm into each egg for ICSI.

Fertilisation Day and Onwards

On the day after the egg collection, the embryologist will call all patients to report the fertilisation rates. A 'good' fertilisation rate is generally thought to be around 70% so from 10 eggs we usually expect about 7 fertilised. This figure is, of course, an average and it will vary from person to person depending on the egg and sperm quality. It is possible that no eggs at all fertilise and this is referred to as 'failed fertilisation'. This is relatively rare, but it does exist and if you are unfortunate enough to suffer failed fertilisation then this will be the end of the treatment cycle. This is a sad fact of life and does not mean that the clinic has done something 'wrong'. In this sad event, patients should receive considerable support from the clinic to deal with the immediate bad news and also with the 'next steps' in their treatment. Patients should not be rushed into a second treatment cycle. They should be given time to recover and to consider if they want to proceed either with another IVF treatment cycle or with alternative options such as adoption.

Sometimes there are also eggs which seem to show good signs of fertilisation but do not develop any further. Once again, this is relatively rare but something you should understand. At least 90% of those eggs which show clear signs of fertilisation should begin to divide to form embryos in the days to come.

The embryos will be kept in the laboratory for up to 5 days and during that time, patients should receive regular updates from the embryologists about the progress and perceived quality of the embryos. I say perceived quality of the embryos because in almost all cases (including those patients who are unfortunate enough to pay for time lapse video of their embryos), the quality of the embryos is determined solely by their visual appearance. At present, there is no technology or 'test' which can identify either a 'good' or a 'bad' embryo. This may be available in the future and is discussed later in this book. Equally a 'good' embryo has many steps to complete before it produces a live birth so once again, it is clear that a 'good' embryo is interesting and encouraging but it is not a sign of definite success.

Experience has taught me that a 'good looking embryo' is not necessarily an embryo which will go on to form a pregnancy. This is because there are many more variables to establishing a pregnancy than just the appearance of the embryo. I have, in fact, seen embryos which look 'bad' go on to from a perfectly normal pregnancy. The basic message here is to not give the appearance of your embryos too much status or else you may be very disappointed. It is important but is by far not the only thing which results in a pregnancy.

Embryo Replacement (Transfer) Day

This is arguably the most exciting and interesting day for most fertility patients. You will get to see your embryos and to begin the next phase of your treatment. You may notice that I prefer to call this process replacement and not transfer. This is because the tradition at Bourn Hall Clinic was to call it replacement and I like tradition. It also seems to make more sense to talk about replacement which to me infers a returning of something to its natural or normal place, where transfer to me refers to moving something from one place to another. Whatever the terminology (as Shakespeare said, a rose by any other name would smell just as sweet) you will get one or two great looking embryos placed back into your uterus and this is the potential start of a pregnancy! Most clinics now offer a photograph of the embryo which has been replaced. Please take time to relax and enjoy the embryo replacement procedure as much as possible.

It's Freezing in Here!

You will also find out at embryo replacement day whether or not any embryos are suitable to freeze. This judgement of suitability to freeze is once again based on visual appearance but in this case embryos which look 'bad' before freezing have been shown to do very badly when thawed out for a later frozen embryo transfer. Embryologists can therefore make a better evidence-based decision on freezing. If you do get some embryos frozen (you might hear some embryologists refer to vitrification, this is just a type of freezing commonly used today) then this potentially gives you a 'reserve' of embryos to use in the future if the current embryos do not form a pregnancy or if a pregnancy and delivery results then the frozen embryos will be a source of potential siblings. Embryos are frozen in liquid nitrogen at -196°C and can be stored for at least 10 years. This reserve of frozen embryos will hopefully allow you to create your required family. It is however worth remembering that not all frozen embryos survive the thawing process and the live birth rate from frozen embryo replacement is 30-35% at best.

Pregnancy Test Day

Fourteen days after your egg collection (the so called 'two-week wait') you will be asked to carry out a pregnancy test to see if the treatment cycle has created an early pregnancy. Most patients do this at home and report the result back to the clinic. There are of course 2 possible option here: pregnant or not pregnant.

If you find that the test shows that you are pregnant at this stage, then this can be an enormous relief for patients. This is true with one little bit of additional advice which the clinic should give. This is a simple reminder that this is a very early pregnancy and there is a long, long way to go to a live birth. Despite this, a positive result at this early stage is a million times better than a negative result.

In the event of a negative result, the clinic will advise on next steps and support you through this difficult time. Some patients feel quite depressed at this stage especially when the cost and stress of getting to this point can be considerable. This is why, it is very important to always have in your mind that the pregnancy and live birth rate for IVF is 30%. I don't say this to be negative but just to be realistic. Having inflated expectations of success, having been told at replacement that your embryos and everything else 'looks great', is a bad thing in a process with a 30% success rate. Try to stay objective and rational in the event of a negative pregnancy test and remember that a frozen embryo replacement may be a possibility in the future or if not another treatment cycle. The main thing is not to rush into anything. I suggest at least one month off between treatment cycles, preferably longer.

The Day 35 'Heart Beat Scan'

Thirty-five days after your egg collection and a positive pregnancy test the next 'hurdle' is a scan to establish if there is a fetus with a heartbeat present in your uterus. The fertility clinic will carry out this scan for you. This may be a very stressful time in the process. If a heartbeat is found, then this is considered to be an 'established' pregnancy and your care will continue with the maternity team at your local hospital in the same way as in a natural conception all the way to delivery of your baby. A heartbeat at this early stage does not necessarily mean that there will be a normal live birth, but it is certainly one more step towards your goal.

If the heartbeat cannot be found at this scan, then this can be devastating news for the patients. The delight and optimism of the positive day 14 pregnancy test may seem irrelevant and cruel. Patients will receive all of the support needed by the fertility clinic and other healthcare professionals. There may have to be surgical removal of the 'products of conception' from the uterus and your clinic will advise you and support you through this process. This procedure, if needed, usually takes place in your local hospital.

KEY POINTS OF CHAPTER 9

- The IVF 'journey' will have many ups and downs and may not result in the outcome you are looking for.

- Do not be 'fast-tracked' into IVF. Your clinic should give you the time and opportunity to explore all options before starting an IVF treatment cycle.
- Time is often short in female fertility treatment; if this is the case, then faster action may be needed to optimise the outcome.
- Egg collection day is a stressful time for many fertility patients, seek additional support from your clinic if needed.
- Fertilisation is the next big step, along with the perceived 'quality' of embryos.
- Embryo replacement day should be as relaxed as possible, you may even get a photograph of your embryo.
- Some embryos may be suitable to freeze but it is not unusual for none of the remaining embryos being suitable to freeze.
- The positive day 14 pregnancy test and Day 35 ultrasound scan are big hurdles which only 30% of patients at best achieve. Think about the importance of managing your own expectations in these very early days of pregnancy.

CHAPTER 10

Advice to Fertility Patients

Peter Hollands

(Advice on Treatments, Clinics and many other Things)

> *Advice is like snow - the softer it falls, the longer it dwells upon, and the deeper it sinks into the mind.*
> **Samuel Taylor Coleridge**

Summary: This chapter helps to dispel some of the myths surrounding fertility treatment and to provide some hopefully welcome advice. It covers the excellent, reliable advice which may be provided by healthcare professionals along with some not so good advice (positive and negative) which may be very disruptive to the overall mood of all fertility. This can result in creating either false hope or false gloom and both of these are potentially very damaging. Advice should be factual, truthful, honest and based on the best information available. Any other forms of advice just cause worry, stress and even potentially depression. Fertility patients must be very selective about the advice they seek and view it all with a critical and well-informed eye.

INTRODUCTION

This is arguably the most important chapter in this book and a chapter which many readers might read in isolation. I would suggest that the chapter is read in the context of the rest of the book because this will make it more understandable and useful. Fertility patients (as most other types of patients) crave advice, and this can make them very vulnerable and easily stressed or anxious. Good advice will help you through the process; bad advice will make the process more stressful and even possibly unsuccessful.

Fertility patients 'consume' an enormous amount of advice during their experience of IVF. This is possibly more than any other patient undergoing other treatments. There will be the obvious fertility clinic healthcare professionals providing advice who are fully qualified physicians, nurses and clinical embryologists. This may take the shape of both verbal and written advice. Take special notice of written advice; it is provided for a very specific purpose. This purpose is that many studies have shown that all types of patients, especially stressed patients, often do not 'hear' or fully comprehend verbal advice. If the patients can go away and quietly read about what was said, then the overall understanding and comprehension are greatly improved. The advice from a fertility clinic is solid, factual and reliable advice (most of the time). The advice may not be what you want to hear but if it comes from healthcare professionals, it should hopefully be true and reliable. It is, however, extremely sad that I have to use the words 'should hopefully' in the previous sentence. There is sadly some advice coming out of some IVF clinics (for example, advice related to add-ons including ICSI) which may be very unreliable and even be deliberately misleading. This puts the onus on the fertility patient to work out what to believe and what not to believe. This is a very unsatisfactory situation but a disappointing fact of life in current IVF. I hope that this situation changes in the future, but at present, there seems to be no appetite for change either in IVF clinics or by fertility patients. Perhaps the regulatory authorities will step in, or perhaps 'patient power' will begin to dominate where patients will be neither vulnerable nor gullible. Such resources as this book may help fertility patients in this context, but it is a sad state of affairs that some private IVF clinics may lie to patients to achieve increased profitability. This is a very poor practice but sadly, it is common throughout IVF globally at present, possibly because of the 'profit focus' in most fertility clinics. Then there may be friends and family giving 'advice' who often may mean well but could be the source of incorrect and possibly damaging advice. This is sadly even worse if the advice comes from friends and family who may have had success in their own fertility treatment. In this case, the advice often goes along the lines of "We did x, y and z in our treatment and it worked!". Needless to say, this type of anecdotal device is both meaningless and potentially damaging, even if it is well-meaning. What happened to someone else is extremely unlikely to happen to you. Please ignore this advice. I know that this is a difficult thing to ask, but in the long term you will benefit.

MORE ADVICE ON ADVICE

All of these different types of advice, from so many sources, may also increase stress felt by fertility patients which is not helpful at all when being treated for infertility. Then there is the landmine of the internet and social media 'experts' offering 'advice'. Fertility patient 'chat rooms' can be equally disruptive. Especially when people for whom IVF has been successful post contributions or when people post complaints or criticisms about a clinic, or a staff member, which may be the clinic or person you think is actually quite good. The problem with the 'successful' patient posts is not their personal success but they often 'advise' other patients based on their own experience. Such 'electronic' anecdotal advice is often completely wrong and can be extremely damaging to fertility patients in terms of their mood and stress levels. It may also be too optimistic which is equally damaging in the event of a failed treatment cycle. The problem with the negative comments about a clinic or a member of staff at a clinic is that the comments are circumstantial and therefore totally irrelevant to your own experiences which may very well be just the opposite.

Optimism and Electronic Advice

Optimism in life in general and in fertility treatment is a good thing but over-optimism (sometimes called excessive expectations or badly managed expect-ations) is bad. Being over optimistic makes you very vulnerable to significant disappointment because you will have convinced yourself that everything will be perfect, and when it is not, then this will be a much harder blow. The best way to modulate your optimism is to be as well-informed as possible about your treatment by listening as closely as possible in the clinic and carefully reading and understanding any written material provided by the clinic. It is worth noting that the written material provided by the fertility clinics has usually been inspected by the regulatory authorities which should make it is as clear and reliable as possible.

My advice on electronic advice is to try to ignore all 'electronic' informal advice unless it comes from trusted sources such as Regulatory Authorities (*e.g.*, the UK HFEA) or from trusted organisations such as the NHS or the National Institute for Health and Care Excellence (NICE). This is a big thing to ask in this modern electronic world but if you value your sanity, it is worth considering. The pressure and stress generated by getting involved in electronic discussions and worse still, un-moderated electronic advice will do nothing to help you in your fertility treatment. There are far too many people out there trying to promote themselves as some sort of fertility expert or 'guru'. This may be for monetary gain, but it may also be just to promote themselves or even for 'fun'. Please be very critical of these people and, if possible, ignore them completely.

Clinic Counsellor

Every fertility clinic should provide an independent counsellor who is available to speak to all patients being treated in the clinic. These counsellors can advise on all aspects of fertility treatment and, at the same time, can ensure and advise on optimal mental health during what is a very stressful process. The problem in most fertility clinics is that the counsellors are often barely consulted at all by fertility patients. There are some possible reasons for this. Perhaps the modest additional fee charged by counsellors deters some patients? Considering the overall cost of fertility treatment, I find this very hard to believe. Perhaps the term 'counsellor' puts some patients off? I have often heard the phrase "we don't need counselling!" from fertility patients who sometimes seem to see the suggestion that they might find speaking to the counsellor useful some sort of insult. The fact is that clinic counsellors are grossly underused and misunderstood part of IVF and the people who suffer from are fertility patients. The truth is that clinic counsellors are highly experienced, effective and most importantly independent healthcare professionals who are grossly underused.

This problem could be solved by one simple change. This simple change would be to drop the title 'counsellor' and replace it with 'unbiased advisor' or 'fertility advice professional' or anything which does not carry the stigma which some people associate with 'counsellors'. Would any fertility patient become insulted by the suggestion that speaking to an unbiased advisor or fertility advice professional might be useful? I think not. I also think that the potential benefits to the patients would be immense.

I would ask every fertility patient to re-think their views on the services of clinic counsellors. They are extremely important to your general well-being and possibly to the overall success of your fertility treatment. Ignore the title, and benefit from their expertise of counsellors; they are a great resource to you.

Who to Tell?

Many fertility patients struggle to decide who they should tell about their plans to undergo fertility treatment. The primary driver behind this may be that fertility patients feel a certain level of embarrassment about their planned treatment. This should not be the case. Infertility is just another medical condition; it is no more embarrassing than pneumonia or a broken leg. There is no perfect answer to this question of who to tell because it is really a judgement call for each person. My experience of this subject, after having spoken to thousands of fertility patients over the years, is that there are 3 main groups who may, or may not, need to know about your fertility treatment plans. These are family, friends, and work.

Family?

Whether or not to tell family members about plans to undergo fertility treatment is a matter of personal choice based on the relationship that a fertility patient has with different family members. Some family members may be supportive, but at the same time they can be 'over interested' or worse still controlling in the treatment process and ask repeated unwelcome questions about progress and success. How is your stimulation going? How many embryos did you get? Are you pregnant yet? Why didn't it work? Are you starting another treatment cycle? You really have more things to think about than these distracting but perhaps well-meaning questions. This is potentially a source of additional stress to the fertility patient which is best avoided if possible. Please also remember that if you were trying for a baby 'naturally' then you would not discuss the details with your family. It would be between you and your partner and perhaps this is how IVF should be.

Despite all of this, if the family member can be relied upon to be discreet, not to ask too many questions and to be a source of support, not criticism, then this may be the perfect situation. I have found that female patients often confide in their mother and this usually works if the mother has the important values and mind-set mentioned above. They often do but not always. I have found that most male patients seem to take fertility treatment in their stride and do not necessarily need to confide in family members. This, of course, may just be the 'macho' approach of the male who, in general, do not want to explore their hopes, fears and worries. This can be a big problem for some men but as it is difficult for them to ask for help and support than in general, they do not get the help and support they need. If you are a male fertility patient and are struggling with the fertility treatment process in any way, please discuss it with your partner, a family member, a counsellor, or a staff member in your fertility clinic. Do not just keep it to yourself; this might be the manly thing to do, but it is also a very stupid thing to do.

Friends?

Sadly, real life interactions with friends do not always follow the supportive and amusing situations seen in the 1980's sitcom Friends. In terms of sharing fertility treatment experiences with friends, then in general this may be helpful by giving you someone to talk to who will truly listen. The other side of the coin is that a friend may be opinionated or 'know' about fertility or equally, they might be very negative with no real foundation for their negativity. Worse still they might have looked up infertility on the internet, this unfortunately is the most likely option. It is, of course, for the fertility patient to judge whether or not to confide in friends. My observation would be to be very selective and to use caution about the content and extent of information shared with friends. Your true friend in the fertility treatment process is your partner. This is the best person in whom to confide and trust.

Should I Tell People At Work?

Almost all fertility patients I have come across over the years (male and female) have full-time employment at the time of their fertility treatment. This means that there is a potential source of stress (remember stress and infertility are a bad combination) when fertility patients need to attend the clinic for consultations, scans, blood work, egg collection, embryo replacement and a similar cycle for frozen embryos apart from egg collection. The hard fact is that you will need to take time out of work, sometimes with little or no notice, to achieve what you want to do in your fertility treatment. This will apply more to the female patient than the male, but the male should ideally support his partner as much as possible during the treatment cycle. There are two possible solutions to this:

1. Take annual leave for the whole of your treatment cycle (this is probably unadvisable to most patients because most of the time they will just sit around worrying about their treatment) or

2. Tell a trusted manager (who will keep the information strictly confidential) at your place of work what you are doing and how this will impact your availability to work. If you do this, be realistic. If you need 2 hours to go to a scan appointment and get back to work, then tell them that. Do not try to underestimate or try to make it 'look better', this will just put more stress on you. This approach will take a lot of stress off you and will enable the employer to understand why you are not at work when you should be.

A very popular phrase often used today is to 'manage expectations'. By clearly telling your employer about what you are doing manages their expectations about you during your treatment cycle. If you are unfortunate enough to have an employer who will not consider any flexibility at all during your treatment cycle, then either take unpaid leave or resign. They are not worth the hassle.

Smoking, Alcohol, Obesity and Underweight

Many patients who find they are infertile often realise, or are told, that it is their life-style and life-choices which are contributing to, and sometimes actually causing, their infertility. This may be a shock to hear, and many fertility patients choose to ignore these problems if they exist. Many fertility clinics also choose to simply ignore these problems when they arise in their patients and take them straight to an expensive IVF treatment cycle. This is bad management of these patients who are then using an expensive high technology hammer to crack a very life-style associated nut. This expensive hammer is also very likely to fail.

Smoking

It is a very well-established medical fact that smoking is very bad for the general health and is indeed the direct cause of many deadly diseases such as lung cancer. The toxins which are inhaled during smoking affect every cell in the body, including eggs and sperm and the cells which form the uterus. Smoking is actively discouraged during pregnancy and should be actively discouraged by all fertility clinics prior to fertility treatment. In general terms, most fertility clinics do ask potential patients to stop smoking but they very rarely, if ever, follow this up and provide support to their patients to stop smoking. It is also important to note that both male and female patients should stop smoking. Some patients (mostly male) think that smoking does not affect their fertility. They are wrong. It is unlikely that stopping smoking alone will result in a return to fertility, but it will certainly improve the overall health of anyone and may well contribute to some increase in fertility. If one partner still smokes, then there is also the problem of 'passive' smoking in the non-smoking partner. If either or both of you are smokers and are considering fertility treatment, then please stop smoking ideally several months before your first consultation at a fertility clinic.

Alcohol

Probably one of the most commonly abused intoxicating substances in modern life is alcohol. It is readily available, it is an integral part of many social events and it is a part of normal daily life for some people. The abuse of alcohol may be in the form of excessive 'social' drinking (binge drinking), excessive drinking in private or chronic (*i.e.*, constant) drinking over a long period of time which is not necessarily excessive but constant. This is not helped by the conception that alcohol will help someone to relax and even invigorate people. It does not, alcohol is a poison and it intoxicates. There are even regular claims, sometimes from apparently reliable sources, that certain alcohol (very often red wine) in moderation may be beneficial. The problem here is the word moderation which is difficult to both define and to achieve. Those people who are taking in too much alcohol quite often do not recognise or accept the fact and are equally reluctant to do anything to solve what they see as 'no problem'. The psycho-social interpretation of alcohol being harmless and even beneficial is the source of many problems in society. Alcohol is implicated in approximately 40% of violent crime in addition to increased alcohol associated public disorder, anti-social behaviour and domestic abuse. Up to 35% of deaths on our roads are attributable to excess blood alcohol in drivers. These are clearly major social and health impacts caused by alcohol and they are shocking but at the same time beyond the scope of this book.

In terms of fertility, the basic advice to both male and female patients is to abstain from alcohol during the treatment cycle and of course, for the female to always abstain from alcohol during pregnancy. Ideally, fertility patients should abstain from alcohol for several months before planned fertility treatment. If it is not possible for some reason to abstain from alcohol during the treatment cycle, and I am not sure what this reason may be, then the advice is moderation and certainly no binge drinking. If fertility patients have problems with alcohol consumption, then they should seek further support and advice from their GP. The biggest hurdle here is to admit that a problem exists with alcohol. Most alcoholics exist in a world of denial. Once this has been aired and accepted then the solutions can sometimes be relatively easy. Stopping drinking excess alcohol may possibly result in a return of fertility with no other intervention.

Obesity

Probably one of the worst social and medical problems in the developed world is obesity. It is estimated that there are approximately 2 billion obese people in the world and that the prevalence of obesity is rising most sharply in children. This is a biological time bomb waiting to explode. Obesity pre-disposes people to heart attack, cancer, stroke and diabetes, as described below. Most people in most developed countries seem blind to the problem. It is known that obesity contributes significantly to the development of heart disease and cancer which are the two top causes of death in the world. It is also associated with the development of diabetes which can result in the loss of vision, limbs and life. If you are male or female and are obese, then it is good general advice to try to reduce your obesity. If you are male or female and infertile and obese then reducing your obesity alone could be a major step towards the return of fertility.

Female Obesity

In female fertility, patient obesity is associated with anovulation (failure to ovulate), poor embryo quality and poor quality of the endometrium into which embryos have to implant. This means that an obese female fertility patient has three extremely important problems which will directly and repeatedly result in infertility if obesity persists. If such a person does manage to become pregnant, then the obesity may then result in an increased rate of miscarriage and more potential problems with the baby at the point of birth. When all of these problems are considered, along with the increased risk of cancer, stroke, heart disease and diabetes, it would seem sensible for the infertile female to try to reduce her weight. This is the advice which is almost always given to obese patients attending an IVF clinic, but it is advice which is very rarely heeded by the patient for a variety of reasons. These may be that the patient does not understand (or even accept) that they are obese, and that this obesity is contributing to their infertility. I have even heard suggestions that IVF clinics are discriminating against obese patients and comments such as "my sister is fat, and she has got 2 kids!" have been heard to ring around fertility clinics many times. Both of these thoughts are nonsense. I have already mentioned in detail that anecdotal reports of fertility in someone else do not mean that these reports have any validity at all to another different patient (even a sister). Regarding IVF clinic discrimination against obese patients, I find this very hard to believe on the basis that the whole focus of an IVF clinic is to get patients onto treatment cycles to make money. IVF clinics do, however, have to follow regulatory advice on the maximum weight of patients they are allowed to treat. Clinically obese patients cannot be treated. Despite this, the IVF clinics do not offer any support to reduce obesity but are still keen to get an obese patient onto a treatment cycle if at all possible. In most IVF clinics, female patients need to have a body mass index (BMI) between 19 to 30, according to the regulatory guidance. The means that the 'ideal' weight for a female IVF patient, of an average height of 5 feet 5 inches, is from 118lbs (8.5 stone) to 186lbs (13 stone). Anything above *or below* this range has a major impact on your fertility. If a patient is obese, then there is no magic formula, milk shake, tablet or diet which will result in weight loss. Weight loss requires willpower and determination which are things a fertility patient should have plenty. The basic premise for weight loss is to take **regular exercise**, eat smaller portions, no 'snacks' **at all** at any time, eat less fat and sugar (including high sugar soft drinks) and consume less or no alcohol. In cases of severe obesity, there are surgical procedures which may help, but this must not be seen as a route to weight loss for fertility treatment. This is usually only considered when obesity is so bad that it may result in death.

Underweight Patients

If a female is under-weight, then this can have just as significant effect on her fertility as being overweight. An under-weight female (BMI less than 19) will often have erratic periods or sometimes even no periods at all. This obviously has a major impact on her fertility. Compared to obesity, it is relatively rare to see an under-weight female patient at fertility but over the years, I have known of a few and they all needed considerable support. First of all, it is very important to exclude any underlying disease which may be the reason for the low weight. This will need other investigations outside the fertility clinic. Then if this is clear, then the psycho-social situation of the patient should be explored, and this is yet another area where the counsellor may be useful. The patient will need to gain weight before any fertility treatment can proceed and this may, of course, result in a return of natural fertility. The extreme position in under-weight patients is that of anorexia nervosa and bulimia nervosa. These are both life-threatening diseases and anyone who think that they might be suffering from either should seek medical help immediately. The problem, of course, is that such patients often do not see that they have a problem and sometimes fiercely resist help. This is where friends, family and ultimately healthcare professionals can be the difference between life and death.

If a male patient is under-weight, then the production of sperm may be severely reduced, and the ability of the sperm produced to fertilise may also be reduced. The management of this is the same as that for the female patient and it poses the same very serious implications to his well-being and life.

Male Obesity

In the male patient, obesity has a similarly high impact on fertility. Obesity in the male has just the same general health implications as in the female and it can be just as damaging to male infertility. In terms of male fertility, if the male is obese then it has been shown that this reduces testosterone (the key male hormone) levels which can result in a reduction in the number and quality of sperm created in the testes. This can lead directly to infertility. There is also good evidence that obesity can result in erectile dysfunction which in turn leads to infertility.

The 'ideal' weight for a male IVF patient of about 5 feet 10 inches tall is from 133lbs (9.5 stone) to 209lbs (15 stone). Any heavier or any lighter than these general guidelines may result in some form of infertility. If the male patient is obese, and he reduces his obesity to a weight in the normal range, then it is highly likely that this will have a beneficial effect on fertility. The method by which weight can be managed and regulated is exactly the same as that described for the female above.

It is important that both the male and female partners treat obesity seriously, not only for their fertility but also for their ongoing general health. A good IVF clinic will recognise this problem and support the patients in their quest to lose weight.

Back-to-Back Treatment Cycles

Once a couple joins the fertility treatment 'treadmill' there is increasing pressure to get as many treatments as possible completed with the perception that this will maximise the possibility of a positive outcome. This is incorrect. Treatment cycles must be measured in quality not quantity. There is also the perception by older female patients that time is 'running-out' and that it is extremely urgent to get as many treatments as possible before natural fertility fades away. This is correct in that female fertility declines dramatically beyond the age of 40. The problem here is more related to society and life-style than biology. Many women today want a career before a family. This is fine but there is sadly a compromise in this thinking which may not always be totally obvious to the patients. The problem is that if a woman leaves trying to become pregnant until she is late 30's or even early 40's and then discovers a problem with her fertility then the chances of success following fertility treatment is on the decline to the point where even the best chances of success are in low single figures. Some people will suggest that egg freezing could be the answer to this problem, but this may not be the case and it is discussed in detail below. When a patient realises that they may be infertile and that 'time may be running out' there then follows a 'panic' for treatment cycles which may result in 'back-to-back' treatment cycles. This is when a couple have a failed treatment cycle and then go ahead with another treatment immediately after the failed cycle. This places considerable physical and mental stress on the patients. The fertility clinics will be happy to accommodate these demands for 'back-to-back' treatment cycles because it maximises patient throughput and therefore profit.

In general terms 'back-to-back' treatment cycles are a bad idea for the patient and for the overall chance of success. The body of the female patient needs a break from the considerable demands of an IVF treatment cycle and both male and female patients need a break from the considerable psychological demands of an IVF treatment cycle. The 'vicious cycle' then appears that the female patient is older, and she feels that the amount of time available to her for a successful treatment cycle is declining and therefore treatment cannot wait. A gruelling and expensive series of 'back-to-back' fertility treatments follow which inevitably result in failure.

I can hear some people crying out 'I got pregnant aged 41 using IVF, this is not a problem!'. Sadly, this kind of result is the exception, not the rule. Any woman who lets herself believe that she can delay having a family with little or no risk of failure is sadly misinformed and misled.

The real-world answer to this conundrum is that women must be more aware about what is possible and what is not possible. If they choose to delay even thinking about having children before their late 30's to early 40's then it must be clear to them that if any problems at all arise, and that even with high technology 'back-to-back' fertility treatments, the chance of a live birth resulting is vanishingly low. This is another tough fact, but I make no apologies for making the point. This subject cannot be buried in the sand and we all hope that it will go away. It must be faced up to if we are to solve this problem in modern socio-biology.

Egg Freezing: Good Idea, False Hope or Money-Making Machine?

Following on from the rather alarming discussion above about the 'fertility clock' slowing and stopping for some women just when they want a family, we now have to consider the relatively new phenomenon of egg freezing. The possibility of freezing eggs is relatively new technology. It raises the possibility of a woman freezing her eggs when young and using them later to create a family. There are some very important points which need to be clarified about this process.

First of all, if a young woman wants to freeze her eggs to use 'later' then this will require ovarian stimulation as described earlier followed by ultrasound guided egg collection. This may not sound like it, but this is the easy bit. The next step is the egg freezing itself. This requires removal of the cells surrounding the egg which first of all means that if the eggs are thawed and fertilised later (which is the basic plan) then ICSI must be used. Let's assume that a woman freezes her eggs when she is 25 years old and wants to use them to start a family when she is 37 years old. In theory we have an older woman who effectively has younger eggs, so far so good!

The next step in the process is to thaw the eggs. Let's assume that the woman had 15 eggs frozen. How many of these 15 eggs should be thawed? In most countries, our imagined patient can only receive a maximum of 2 embryos. Following discussion with the patient, it is decided to initially thaw 4 eggs. All of them fail to thaw. Another 4 eggs are thawed, and 2 eggs survive. These are both injected with her partners sperm and 2 embryos suitable for replacement are created. So far so good.

The problem which now arises, and there is no known solution apart from a time machine, is that we have embryos from 'young' eggs going into a woman whose natural fertility and ability to carry a pregnancy has declined over the years. The uterus, endometrium and reproductive hormones in the proposed mother are all on the decline. All worries are confirmed when the pregnancy test comes back negative. In a final attempt the woman thaws the remaining eggs and following ICSI two embryos develop which are replaced. The pregnancy test is positive, but an early miscarriage follows, and the pregnancy is lost. The point which I am trying to make here is that egg freezing when young does not guarantee that a pregnancy and live birth can be achieved when older. It is possible but it most certainly is not guaranteed. Everyone involved must understand this.

The other problem with egg freezing is that it is very profitable for fertility clinics and is therefore marketed very strongly despite the drawbacks outlined above. Patients should remember that it is not only the initial cost of the egg freezing which in the UK is £3500-£4500 (at least 50% of this is profit) but also the annual storage fee for the frozen eggs which is £200-£360 (at least 90% of this is profit). If a fertility clinic stores frozen eggs for 500 patients (this could easily be done by a large clinic with excellent if not exactly ethical marketing) then this could result in £1.75 to £2.25 million in immediate income for the egg freezing and an annual income of £100,000 to £180,000 which is almost all straight profit for 10 years or more. This would be a total potential income of at least £1 to £1.8 million from the storage fees alone. This enormous cost and profit may seem acceptable if the process could reliably restore fertility to older women but as described above it does not. It would be much cheaper, easier and reliable to decide to have a baby by age 30 at the latest.

Another variation on this theme proposed by some is to suggest that the young frozen eggs once fertilised could be replaced into a young surrogate mother. This scenario would make the establishment of a pregnancy and a live-birth much more likely, but the cost of the procedure, not to mention the emotional detachment, might not be as welcome. Egg freezing is interesting technology, but it is not some sort of miracle answer to the conundrum of reproduction for the career woman. Anyone who tells you otherwise is almost certainly a marketing man.

Add-ons

A previous chapter in this book has dealt with the subject of add-ons in fertility treatments in detail. Patients are well advised to resist the temptation of add-ons because they are untested and unproven and as such will *not help in any way* in terms of increasing the live-birth rate for any patient. The only other bit of advice on add-ons to patients is that it is worth keeping a close watch on the developments in add-on technology which as of today is very poor, but in the future might improve to the point where certain add-ons *might* become useful. This is an ever-changing field. Such future developments would have to be based a clinical trial of the technology in question which showed a clear benefit to patients from the add-on which was tested. This is something which can be used as part of your questioning of fertility clinics about 'add-ons'.

Pregnancy, Birth and Parenthood

It is beyond the scope of this book to provide detailed information and advice on pregnancy, birth and parenthood, but it is a good place to bring these subjects to mind so that fertility patients can understand the basics and be prepared for what might come.

Fertility patients have a complete focus on their goal of achieving a pregnancy and a subsequent live-birth. They have considerable emotional, physical and financial commitment to the process, which they fully understand (or hopefully fully understand) has a low success rate but at the same time, if it works, can potentially bring much joy and happiness both for the parents and for the family. It may therefore come as a surprise when some patients find that pregnancy, childbirth and parenthood is perhaps not the happy, enjoyable experience which they had anticipated it to be. The best way to approach pregnancy, childbirth and parenthood is to understand the potential problems which may arise at the various stages. It is also a good idea to have in mind what can be done to help you if needed. Some fertility patients may also have a 'rosy' image of pregnancy, childbirth (also known as labour for a good reason) and parenthood. This is not a bad thing *per se,* but it is certainly worth spending a few moments considering the implications of becoming a parent in the harsh light of day.

Pregnancy

Pregnancy involves considerable changes in the female body, the female physiology and often the emotional mind-set of the woman. Some women find these changes acceptable and part of the process, other may find them very distressing. It is probably not wise to dwell on every possible complication of pregnancy because this would just cause unnecessary anxiety for most people. The important thing to keep in mind is that there will be physical and emotional changes during and after pregnancy and that these will be different for all women. There is considerable support for pregnant women from GPs and midwives during pregnancy and all pregnant women should seek medical advice and assistance if needed.

Childbirth (Labour)

Once again, the subject of childbirth or labour is well out of the scope of this book, but it is an inevitable and welcome consequence of a successful fertility treatment cycle, so it is certainly worth a few moments consideration. I have two insights into childbirth (this is actually a strange term because a baby is born, not a child!) from the male point of view. One as a healthcare professional working in a delivery unit and secondly as a father-to-be. As a healthcare professional, childbirth is a relatively relaxed and controlled atmosphere with periods of rapid and sometimes life-saving activity. As a father-to-be, it ranged from relaxed to highly stressed, from worried to exhausted, from optimistic to just wishing it would all soon be over, and finally to utmost relief that both mother and baby came through the whole process intact. Every father will relate to these feelings.

The female, of course, has a more 'hands-on' role to play in childbirth. She has to endure pain, discomfort and medical and sometimes surgical interventions which can be life threatening both to her and the baby. It is a physical and emotional rollercoaster which marks the start of a whole new phase in the life of the mother and baby. The mother may come away from experience with many stitches and even haemorrhoids as a souvenir of the big event. She also may suffer 'baby blues' in the days following birth of a baby which for most women is transient and, whilst unpleasant, it is something which most women can endure. If the 'baby blues' go on for a longer time, and the mood of the mother stays very low, then this can be post-natal depression. This is a much more serious problem and any woman who suspects that she may have post-natal depression should seek medical advice and support immediately. The problem here is that some women do not recognise the problem and it may be for her partner or husband to ask for assistance on her behalf.

There is of course much more to childbirth than this perhaps trivial view. In terms of the fertility patient, and all parents to be, it is important to gain as much knowledge and information as possible and take this life-changing process in your stride as you did with fertility treatment.

Parenthood

I do not claim to be an expert on parenthood in any shape or form. I have two children who have both managed to become adults so from that point of view, I have 'been there and got the T-shirt'. One thing which never changes from my point of view and from that of many other people is that parenthood is forever. When children become adults, the parents still view them as 'their kids'. This can cause unnecessary stress both for the children and the parents if the parent is too controlling. There is no magic answer to good parenthood but the virtues of love, respect, mutual support and money when needed is a good place to start.

A Second Opinion?

As in any branch of medicine, a second opinion is available to all fertility patients. This is sadly something which, in my experience, very few fertility patients pursue. This may be because they fully trust the physician treating them and do not feel that a second opinion is necessary. On the other hand, some patients may feel that seeking a second opinion is in some way questioning the knowledge and ability of their physician and clinic. This is not the case. A second opinion can be refreshing, illuminating, shocking and re-assuring and it might even save a lot of time and money. It might even be the difference between success and failure of your treatment cycle. The best point at which to seek a second opinion is when the diagnosis has been made and a clear treatment plan has been proposed. This will give the person providing the second opinion the chance to review the proposed treatment with a critical mind-set. Such a second opinion will either confirm a sensible treatment plan or it may identify things which are missing, things which are just wrong, things which are just there to increase profit and worst of all, untested and unproven technologies being offered as part of routine treatment.

There are many people who could provide a second opinion, but it is absolutely critical that if you seek a second opinion, then it should be from someone who is appropriately qualified, someone who has respect from their peers and someone who is not a maverick. It does not necessarily have to be someone from a fertility clinic. The person providing a second opinion may be a physician, a clinical embryologist, a fertility nurse or a counsellor (yes, counsellors can and do help) depending on the nature of your concerns or the questions you would like to be answered. A second opinion should cost no more than a first consultation and some people will even give their help and advice for no fee. These are my kind of people!

A second opinion should be part of every fertility treatment cycle. Sadly, it is a very rare event and in normal practice a second opinion is not received until fertility patients switch clinics. They then often find that switching clinics and a second opinion was the best move they ever made. A second opinion may save time and money, it will provide re-assurance to the patients, it will identify any problems with proposed treatment and in doing so may make the primary carer to think again. Most importantly it might be the key to success in your fertility treatment.

CHANGING FERTILITY CLINICS?

It is not rare to hear of fertility patients who have undergone 5-10 treatments (sometimes a lot more!) at the same fertility clinic and spent enormous amounts of money. The fertility patients often say that their rationale for this loyalty may be that the clinic 'know us' or that they 'know our problems' or simply that 'we like this clinic'. This logic does not make any sense at all. If they have had multiple failed treatments at any clinic then surely trying a different approach from someone else might be a good option? If you took your car to a garage and they returned it in a worse state than when it went in, would you then go back to them for more? I think not.

Fertility clinics operate in a very competitive environment. They worry a lot about their live birth rates and will even resort to 'massaging' data to make their live-birth rate look better than it is in reality. The best live-birth rate data to look at is that provided by regulatory authorities for each clinic which is independently audited and reliable. You are a 'customer' in these clinics and if you do not like the service, the people, the surroundings or anything else about the clinics then there are many other clinics who may be able to do a better job and will be very happy to see you. The advice here is do not feel 'tied' to a clinic, you owe them nothing. If I was a patient, I would not stick with one clinic for more than 2 failed treatment cycles. Moving on will allow your case to be viewed by new eyes (this is always a good thing) and the chance for new people to deliver the treatment service they think most appropriate. You might even like the staff at the new clinic!

INFERTILITY AND MENTAL HEALTH

There have been many reports in previous years about the significant decline in mental health in some fertility patients. On the face of it, this is not surprising because fertility treatment is a physical, emotional and financial strain to everyone. Every patient is different in terms of the support they have from their partner, their family, their friends and where relevant their workplace. They all have different financial positions, and some may even have a history of poor mental health stretching back long before infertility was identified. This is a very complex and very important aspect of the overall delivery of fertility treatment which many fertility clinics either ignore or provide inadequate support. It is also important to note that for fertility treatment, we almost always have to consider 2 patients, the obvious exception here are, of course, single women seeking treatment and the extremely rare situation of a single man seeking treatment. This unusual situation of 2 patients per treatment means that the interactions between patients may result in decreasing levels of mental health. An example here is one patient blaming the other for the situation they find themselves in. For the single patients they have the situation where they have to cope with everything without a partner which could be just as stressful.

We must however be clear that there is a very big difference between being stressed and having decreased levels of mental health. Stress might seem all consuming on the day in which it happens but a week later it is ancient history, and the patients are back on an even keel. This is a position which most, if not all, of fertility patients will experience at some point during their treatment. This is not depression.

A depressed patient will have many signs and symptoms beyond the scope of this book but the main thing with depression is that it arises and in time it gets worse, not better. The patient may have a low mood or continual sadness, self-esteem may be reduced (especially where the patient is dealing with previous failed treatment cycles), tearfulness and sometimes guilt may be shown along with irritability and intolerance of others. There may also be a lack of motivation, difficulty in making decisions and being anxious or worried all the time. Not every patient will show every symptom, but these are the main symptoms to be aware of and remember that the patient him/herself might not accept that they are suffering from these problems.

This downward spiral may result in the patient becoming very introspective, non-communicative and even losing interest in the treatment itself. These are major alarm bells and medical advice must be sought immediately. This is easier said than done because depressed patients often claim that they are 'fine' when challenged and state clearly that they do not want to speak to anyone or need any help. In this situation, you may seek initial help and advice from the fertility clinic staff. The fertility clinic counsellor is also a fantastic resource in this context and, as I have mentioned many times, is grossly underused by most fertility patients.

If a depressed fertility patient does not seek help, then things will inevitably get worse with time. Help can come in the form of many things, from medication to talking therapy to counselling, but the key thing is to seek help.

There have been cases where fertility patients have become seriously depressed, have received and sought no help at all and have progressed to the point of considering or attempting suicide. If anyone gets to this stage, then they must go to A&E or call the emergency services immediately. Mental health awareness is thankfully on the increase and Government funding in the UK has increased to provide better mental health services. If you or your partner are suffering from poor mental health then please seek help, do not delay and do not be embarrassed. Your actions could be life-saving.

IVF MYTHS

There are many 'myths' about IVF. Our dear friends on the internet help these myths to proliferate and sometimes even grow to the status of becoming 'true' simply because of the way in which the myths are promoted. Perhaps the most damaging myth in fertility is the idea that the only treatment for infertility is IVF. This has been discussed in detail throughout this book and is clearly incorrect. Infertility may be resolved in many ways and IVF should be the final, not the first, option. It is analogous to an obese patient who goes straight to gastric band surgery without trying dieting, exercise and life-style changes first.

A second damaging myth is that infertility is a woman's problem. Infertility can be a result of a problem with the female, the male or both. It is potentially damaging for either 'blamed' or for it to be a 'woman's problem' even if female infertility is the cause of infertility.

Many of the other myths in IVF are trivial such as fad foods, fad exercise and 'lucky-pants'. These myths are usually harmless and may even be entertaining. As always, keep a clear head and a critical mind and all will be well.

KEY POINTS OF CHAPTER 10

- Advice might be useful, but it is only as good as the person giving the advice.
- Try to be very selective about the electronic 'advice' available, it might not be as reliable or true as you might think.

- Please take advantage of the skill and service provided by your clinic counsellor.
- Think very carefully about who you confide in about your fertility treatment. These choices could make a big difference to your overall experience.
- Avoid smoking and alcohol and reduce obesity to optimise the outcome of your treatment cycle.
- An under-weight patient needs investigation and possibly treatment to restore weight and possibly restore fertility.
- 'Back-to-back' treatment cycles are best avoided if at all possible.
- Egg freezing when young is currently unproven as a method of retaining fertility for older women and should be approached with caution.
- Pregnancy, birth and parenthood should be understood very well by all fertility patients to minimise problems in the future.
- A second opinion on your fertility treatment is not only available but it is also very welcome.
- Changing fertility clinics is always an option and something which may be beneficial to some patients.
- Good mental health is very important for fertility patients and anyone who feels that their mental health is declining or low should seek help.
- There are many myths in IVF; ignore them all!

The Future of IVF

Peter Hollands

(The 'Next Generation' of IVF)

> *Let us put our minds together and see what life we can make for our children.*
> ***Sitting Bull***

Summary: This chapter summarises the possible future of IVF in terms of new technologies and perhaps even a new mindset. IVF is in need of new technology and a renewed mind-set to improve the service provided to patients and also to increase the overall live-birth success rate which has not really improved since 1978. Some of the ideas presented may be a reality shortly, others may take some time and others have no real part to play in the future of IVF but are part of current debate.

INTRODUCTION

Throughout this book, I have been talking about and reflecting on the current practice of IVF and the problems and challenges faced both by patients and by fertility clinics. There are many issues which need to be resolved in IVF clinics, some of them are relatively easy to resolve and some of them either very difficult or even impossible to resolve. Many of these problems arise from greed, complacency, lack of empathy for patients and a simple lack of momentum and motivation in some fertility clinics. The IVF industry is currently in the wilderness, providing an indifferent service, often not listening to criticism and it has very poor communication, interaction and understanding between the patient and the clinic. There are also unrealistic or poorly managed expectations in some patients; this is not the fault of the patients. It is the fault of the clinics. New technology in IVF clinics might solve or reduce some of these problems but in addition, the human mind-set has to change if true benefits are to be achieved. IVF is in crisis and now is time to put it right.

FUTURE TECHNOLOGY

The technology used in IVF in 1978 was manual, laborious, open to errors and mistakes and it relied on considerable and unique expertise from those healthcare professionals who provided the treatment. Examples of that equipment and technology can be seen in an archive in Churchill College, Cambridge University, dedicated to Bob Edwards who was a Fellow of Churchill College. The equipment and technology may look 'dated' in modern terms, but it did the job, and it is interesting to see where we started compared to where we are now. I also attended Churchill College during my time in Cambridge and spent many a happy evening with Bob Edwards at formal Hall (a formal dinner in College) followed by brandy and inspiring conversation about IVF and stem cells. This was the creative, caring, ethical and evidence based atmosphere in which IVF was developed.

In terms of future technology, it is extremely important to think about the basic principles of the original IVF technology developed by Patrick Steptoe, Bob Edwards and Jean Purdy but at the same time to consider future developments which will be truly innovative and incorporate state-of-the-art technology. Such future developments most importantly must result in a sustained increase in the live birth rate following IVF. An improvement in the live birth rate is the 'Holy Grail' of IVF and will only be achieved by revolutionary new technology and a considerable increase of the knowledge base in which IVF operates. It is important to remember that hindsight is easy, and that foresight is extremely difficult, sometimes impossible. In this discussion of the future of IVF, I will introduce some novel ideas and some concepts which may be far ahead of any current thinking. They may never even get close to happening but if we do not hypothesise, then no progress will be made. Bob Edwards was constantly striving to improve the technology he invented to provide a better service to his parents. Some improvements to IVF were made in the late 20th century, but they were mainly refinements of existing technology such as better incubators or better and safer consumables. In the 21st century, we must take a new view on fertility treatment. This may make fertility treatment easier to carry out, cheaper to provide to the patients and be greatly improved in terms of an increase in live birth rate. In a perfect world, all of these things will happen. Sadly, the world is not perfect but most of the present and future scientists and physicians will endeavour to make improvements to IVF.

The Starting Point

In the early 1980's, I was working with Bob Edwards, Patrick Steptoe and Jean Purdy at Bourn Hall Clinic as one of the first ever Clinical Embryologists in the world. These were pioneering and exciting times because the treatment was still very new and there was still much to learn about male and female infertility and how to best handle human embryos in the laboratory. The overall live birth rate in those early days was around 30% when considering all age groups and all diagnoses. This overall live birth rate has not changed since these early days despite the efforts to improve it and despite the fact that some clinics make unsupported claims of 'high' live birth rates. This is purely a marketing scam to attract patients to their clinic. The laboratory technology at Bourn Hall Clinic was entirely manual and all of the reagents and culture media were prepared at Bourn Hall Clinic using starting materials purchased largely from scientific suppliers. The treatment was on a partially inpatient basis with the female patient staying at Bourn Hall for up to 3 weeks during treatment and the male patient living either locally in the village of Bourn or in nearby Cambridge. At this time, it was already possible to freeze human embryos and frozen donor sperm was available if the male had insufficient sperm for *in vitro* fertilisation. It is easy to look back with rose tinted glasses but these early days of IVF in my opinion were the best. The afternoon tea and cakes provided by the chef at Bourn Hall Clinic were also second to none and a welcome respite in a long difficult shift. In addition, there was a true team ethic in place across the whole clinic. Nurses, embryologists and physicians were involved in clinical decision making resulting in a coherent and robust service for patients.

The process of IVF is now on a totally outpatient basis and there are clinics in almost every large town with sometimes, in places such as London, many clinics in one town. Consultations are held at the clinic and most clinics provide 'open evenings' for prospective patients. Female patients visit the clinic for their monitoring scans and blood tests, and they administer their own medication by injection. The egg collection is carried out under light sedation and the patient goes home later that day. She then returns for the embryo replacement and then carries out a home pregnancy test when the time comes to see if the treatment worked. This places a considerable additional burden on the female patients, which we would all do well to carefully think about. Fertility itself is a stressful situation and we may want to think about how this high pressure out-patient service impacts already stressed patients. The role of the male is apparently even less in that he is only actually needed to produce a semen sample on the day of egg collection. The male does, of course, play a considerable and essential role in support of his partner during treatment. Today it is even possible to freeze semen before the treatment cycle and I have been involved in many IVF treatments where the male partner was overseas or elsewhere at the time of the treatment. This detachment of the male and female patient in the treatment process and the demands it puts onto the female patient in particular does nothing for the overall success of the treatment. It also, in my mind, raises possible questions about the level of commitment of such male patients to the treatment process. Should a business meeting or other overseas travel really be more important than supporting your partner during fertility treatment? I would hope that the answer to this question is no.

Everyone agrees that a stressed patient means a patient who is less likely to succeed, and the delivery of modern IVF means that stress levels are potentially high for all patients. In addition, there are patients who attend fertility clinics describing 'infertility' who are immediately placed onto an IVF treatment cycle. No consideration is taken of the general and mental health of the patient or whether or not simple interventions such as weight loss or life-style changes may significantly increase their chances of achieving a natural pregnancy. The drive to go for a high profit IVF cycle is irresistible and this is another area for some serious soul searching by those running IVF clinics.

Innovations

Moving forward in embryology, the next big innovation in IVF was Intracytoplasmic Sperm Injection (ICSI), as described earlier. ICSI was originally developed to help male patients who did not produce enough sperm for IVF and for those patients who had enough sperm for IVF but still suffered failed fertilisation. In this context, ICSI was a great innovation and it was very welcome in this context. The drawbacks of ICSI are that it involves considerable manipulation of human gametes, it requires additional training for clinical embryologists to become competent in the technique and the equipment required for the microinjection is expensive. As a result, when ICSI was offered, it involved a significant extra cost to patients. Those patients did benefit immensely from ICSI, so this extra cost was justified and acceptable. Today ICSI is *the most overused* technique in modern IVF. Many clinics boast that they use ICSI on almost all patients and patients see this as a good thing because of the way in which it is sold to them as a 'guarantee' of fertilisation. This means that patients who have no clinical need for ICSI still undergo invasive ICSI at considerable additional cost. The fertilisation 'guarantee' is also false marketing as it is well known that failed fertilisation is still possible despite using ICSI. The use of medical technology which is not clinically indicated is not allowed in all other areas of clinical practice so why does this happen in IVF? This is like telling someone with an ingrowing toenail that they need a leg amputation!

Profit!

The major problems in IVF today revolve around the development of IVF as a profit-making procedure. There is nothing inherently wrong with this as there are many other private clinics and hospitals offering other treatments for profit. Nevertheless, in IVF there are now thousands of clinics worldwide and some of these are 'mega' clinics who treat thousands of patients *per annum* and generate a massive income for their owners and investors. This income is enhanced considerably in all clinics by the use of ICSI when it is not indicated or needed.

This is unethical and exploitation of vulnerable patients who naturally trust the advice they get from clinics. If we are to make good progress in the future in the treatment of infertility, then this profit orientated mind-set has to change. This might be achieved by new clinic management, new ideas, regulatory changes and improvements and fertility patients with a much clearer understanding of the process who are not afraid to ask difficult questions.

Following on the over-use of ICSI, there are currently many more so called 'add-ons' which are offered to patients to allegedly increase their overall chances of live birth. These were described in detail earlier in this book. There are too many of these 'add-ons' from 'embryo glue' to 'endometrial scratching' but the problem is that none of these 'add-ons' have been proven to be effective. Once again, we have IVF clinics openly exploiting the hopes and fears of fertility patients for profit with no fear of being challenged. Perhaps the most ridiculous and expensive of these 'add-ons' is the 'technology' which involves creating a time-lapse video of embryonic development and then claiming that this video will enable the clinical embryologist to select the 'best' embryo to replace into the mother. The equipment needed to create such a video is extremely expensive and the additional fee to the patients is high. The overall benefit of this technology to live birth rate is zero. This use of 'add-ons' in IVF is a scandal ready to break and when it does, there may be many lawsuits from angry patients who have paid money for pointless procedures and technology.

Stagnation

In my opinion, IVF today has stagnated with no real increase in live birth rate, often an indifferent overall service to patients but ever-increasing profits for clinics. This keeps the business people happy, but this is to the detriment of fertility patients in terms of both the overall quality of their treatment and the cost to the patient. Part of the reason for this may be that some clinics are owned by large corporations and others are run independently by profit focussed businessmen with little thought for fertility patients. Negative patient feedback often reflects this lack of compassion by clinics and some patients are beginning to quite rightly question the ever-increasing cost of treatment along with the apparent decrease in customer service. The only way forward from now on is a complete change in mind-set of those people running IVF clinics to return to ethical, honest practice where nothing is offered unless it has a proven benefit to the patient. All healthcare professionals have a duty of care to their patients which means they should only do things which will benefit the patient. At present in IVF the only people benefitting are the clinics and their investors. This is not the legacy which Edwards, Steptoe and Purdy left us, and it is time that someone spoke out to protect their legacy and to protect patients.

A PROMISING FUTURE?

Despite these dire current problems in IVF, there is an interesting future for IVF. The first thing which needs to happen is a complete revision of the technology used in the embryology laboratory to move away from manual, error prone, procedures to *true* automation. This is not a time-lapse video of a developing embryo. This is technology which can bring together egg and sperm, allow fertilisation, properly monitor this process by assessing the quality and components in the culture media and perhaps using artificial intelligence to decide which are the embryos most likely to form a pregnancy. In addition, we need much more understanding of the process of implantation and how to optimise it to increase the overall live birth rate. Developing new technology for the processing and handling of sperm is also needed. This technology has not really changed since 1978 and it a glaring problem to anyone with even a basic understanding on IVF. This will not mean some sort of automated ICSI. It will mean a new level of understanding on both the physiology and pathology of sperm and a considerable change in the technology used to prepare sperm for IVF.

These and many other developments may bring IVF into the 21st century instead of wallowing in the 20th century. It is also likely that even with perfect embryology, andrology and clinical practice that the success rate of IVF may still not increase. This could be because the success rate we see is that which is defined by nature and no human intervention can change it. If this proves to be true, then patients will have to accept that a 70% failure rate of IVF is to be expected because even the most brilliant minds cannot change things which are inevitable in nature.

The practice of IVF today is at an all-time low because of the factors I have described above. Those providing IVF need to think carefully about the service they are offering and whether or not this service is always in the best interests of their patients. The hard fact is that it is not. Research scientists need to receive the funding and facilities needed to develop new, safe and effective technology for IVF. This needs collaboration between Universities and private clinics and Government support. Edwards, Steptoe & Purdy left us an amazing legacy, my plea is that we do not ruin this legacy by greed, unethical practice and a complete blindness to the future.

Telemedicine

Telemedicine is the remote diagnosis or advice by means of telecommunications technology *i.e.* a mobile phone. The COVID-19 pandemic has resulted in an increased use of telemedicine by GPs and many others and the use of telemedicine is becoming more routine throughout the whole of medical practice. Fertility is no exception and fertility patients can benefit in many ways from the flexibility which telemedicine offers including easier access to physicians, embryologists and nurses for advice, no time and money wasted in travelling to appointments and sitting in the waiting room, less time away from work and family and of course less childcare if the patients already have children. There are also various 'apps' available which can remind patients about medication and can be a useful way of storing such things as blood tests and scan results. Telemedicine of course has limitations, and these are mainly if the patient needs examination, a blood test or scan which clearly cannot be carried out remotely. In the future there will no doubt be many new innovations in telemedicine which will streamline the overall process of fertility treatment.

INVOcell-A Possible Cheaper Version of IVF?

IVF is a costly process. This is because of the technology and facilities needed to deliver IVF treatment and the cost of medication needed by fertility patients. The cost of medication is highly unlikely to change because the owners and investors of these medications will never want to reduce their income for the sake of patients. This is not how big pharma works, profit is king. The only realistic route to making IVF cheaper to provide is by using new, less expensive technology. At present an IVF clinic has to have a fully equipped laboratory, an operating theatre and recovery area, treatment rooms, consulting rooms and administration areas. The provision of these facilities to the approval of the regulatory authorities is a very expensive process. All of this has to be staffed by filly qualified and competent healthcare professionals which is another considerable expense.

One possible solution to the high cost of the IVF laboratory is to use technology such as InvoCell. I should say that I have no connections at all with this company and I do not either recommend or not recommend this company or technology to anyone. It is simply a discussion point which I think is interesting. InvoCell produce a device in which eggs and sperm can be incubated but the difference here is that the incubation takes place in the vagina of the female patient and not in an expensive IVF laboratory. When the embryos are ready to go back into the womb then the device is retrieved by a doctor, the embryos are chosen by an embryologist and the replacement procedure from this point on is exactly the same as that used for all patients. This idea is nothing new. I clearly remember discussions about the possibility of culturing human embryos in this way in the early days at Bourn Hall Clinic. In those discussions the purpose was to possibly improve the fairly primitive culture systems we had available for embryos with a view to perhaps improving embryo quality and overall success rates. The same principle applies today but now the focus is to provide a system which can provide high quality human embryos but at the same time remove the need for an expensive IVF laboratory and pass these savings onto the patient. This sounds perfect but as in most things in life there are imperfections. Some patients may not like the idea of having a culture device fitted into their vagina. Some patients will need ICSI (assuming that they have severe male infertility) and so fertilisation would not take place in the device, but it could still be used for embryo culture. The device may accidentally 'fall out' and the stress of this might be too much for patients to think about. Despite these obvious objections there is certainly still some merit in the technology especially where cost is critical or where the infrastructure simply does not exist for an IVF laboratory. We clearly need to maintain an open mind to these emerging technologies which may help to drive down the cost of IVF to the patient.

Laboratory Automation

The IVF laboratory is a place where great dexterity, focus, skill and attention to detail is needed. There are repetitive procedures which must ideally be carried out with maximum continuity and care no matter what time of day it is or how difficult a shift has been. Clinical Embryologists are consummate professionals but with the best will in the world the repetitive and often physically and mentally tiring procedures carried out in an IVF laboratory will inevitably result in variation of the quality of these procedures. The Clinical Embryologist may be tired, stressed and even bored which results in variation of procedures from patient to patient which in turn results in variable outcomes for similar patients on the same day. This is the current situation, and it is amplified many times when the workload is high.

The answer to achieving consistency and true reproducibility in the IVF laboratory may be automation. When I say automation, I *do not* mean time lapse videos and such nonsense which is currently the fashion in IVF laboratories. Automation means totally new technology which is capable of taking eggs and sperm all the way from insemination to selection of embryos for replacement without any human intervention at all. This is not science fiction and indeed there are many excellent scientists and engineers actively considering this challenge. There also need to be a revolution in ICSI. At present, this is a laborious, intense process which is wide open to operator fatigue and error. Automation of ICSI will be difficult and the initial set-up of the instrument would have to be very precise, but this would result in consistency and accuracy which is impossible when using the current manual system. It would also be nice to see a system which can inject eggs using ICSI and then move them on to automated, undisturbed culture all the way to embryo replacement. Clinical embryologists may complain that such technology would result in considerable de-skilling in their profession, and this is true. De-skilling is an inevitable consequence of automation and advancement in any field, this has been seen throughout clinical diagnostic pathology in the past 40 years and it will no doubt come to clinical embryology. It is also worth noting that Clinical Embryologists did not exist in their current form until 1978 and that their role, responsibility and even existence will no doubt change in the future. The way we do things will always change and improve we see this in everyday life and it will always be that way. In the future, we will see it in the embryology laboratory. The benefit will all go towards the patient and I will be very happy to see that day.

Artificial Intelligence

Artificial intelligence is the use of computer technology to perform tasks normally requiring human intelligence. This may be such things as visual perception, speech recognition and decision-making. Artificial intelligence is slowly being introduced into many areas of clinical practice to improve the efficiency of such things as data analysis and interpretation, for example interpretation of CT/MRI scan results. It can also be used to 'drive' automation as described above and will almost certainly be needed to achieve total automation in IVF.

In terms of fertility treatment, artificial intelligence has many possible applications in such areas as blood test interpretation and ultrasound scan interpretation. These two in parallel would allow decision making on when, what type and how medication should be taken to optimise the patient response. In the laboratory artificial intelligence could assess embryo quality (almost certainly as part of overall automation) and improve semen assessments so that every parameter in a semen analysis is thoroughly assessed for every patient.

Artificial intelligence and automation will go hand in hand in the future and it will be commonplace in the fertility clinic and all other areas of clinical practice of the 22nd century. Once again, the main people to benefit should be the patients although the manufacturers of AI and automation will no doubt also benefit. I have no problem with this as long as any new technology is fully validated and safe and effective to use in fertility treatment.

Quantum Biology and Quantum Physics

You may find it a little strange to find a mention of quantum physics in a book about fertility treatment. This 'coming together' of biology and physics is beginning to create a revolution in our understanding of biological processes and fertility will be no exception.

When I was an undergraduate, I had a great interest in quantum physics even though this was not what I was studying! My interest wandered around the possibility of using quantum physics to describe biology because this could potentially give us the ultimate understanding of both normal health and disease. I asked my life science lecturers about this idea and either usually got a laugh or was told to focus on my subject of natural sciences, not physics. This interest has stayed with me through the years, and it always will.

There have been some very interesting developments in the past 25 years in the field of quantum biology. Quantum biology is the use of quantum physics to describe biological mechanisms and it has already been shown to be useful in adding a total new level of understanding to such things as navigation in birds, vision and photosynthesis (energy production) in plants. In my own research, my colleagues and I have used quantum biology to try to start to understand how laser light interacts with human stem cells and how this can be turned into a potential therapy. In the future I hope to see quantum biology coming into mainstream health care to produce totally new levels of understanding and therapies in clinical medicine.

The science of fertility could potentially benefit from quantum biology because there are so many things which we have yet to fully understand in human reproduction. A detailed quantum understanding of hormone production and action, interactions between egg and sperm, the changes happening in the developing embryo, the quantum mechanism of embryo implantation and the growth of the fetus would revolutionise both understanding and treatment. It will take time, money and committed highly skilled researchers to achieve these ideas but the benefits may be literally beyond our imagination.

PRP and Stem Cells

The use of technology first developed to apply to procedures in regenerative medicine has recently started to be assessed in terms of helping in fertility treatment. The first of these is Platelet Rich Plasma or PRP. PRP is prepared by taking a small amount of peripheral blood and centrifuging it to obtain the part of the plasma (the clear yellow fluid of blood) which contains platelets. PRP treatment is an autologous procedure which means that the PRP is used to treat the same person from which the initial peripheral blood was collected. Platelets are tiny particles in our blood which are involved in the blood clotting process. Platelets can also produce a range of growth factors and messenger chemicals (known technically as cytokines). This makes PRP a potent and concentrated source of growth factors and cytokines which can promote tissue repair and anti-inflammatory action in some situations. PRP is currently used in the treatment of some musculoskeletal diseases such as osteoarthritis of the knee based on the fact that it has anti-inflammatory properties. Patients seem to benefit when PRP is injected directly into the diseased joint although some patients find that the benefits decrease with time and repeat injections are therefore needed for some people PRP has also shown encouraging results in the treatment of patellar tendinopathy and plantar fasciitis.

Patellar tendinopathy is a disease often found in athletes who play jumping sports, and it is caused by the extreme loads which are placed on the knees in such sports resulting in tissue damage and inflammation. Plantar fasciitis is a disease in which there is inflammation of the tissue connecting the heel bone to the toes. It is clear that PRP seems to have a role to play in the treatment of some types of inflammation, but can it be used to treat infertility?

In terms of treating infertility with PRP, there have been some interesting observations that PRP may be able to enhance low ovarian reserve in some women. The PRP was directly injected into the ovary and those patients were compared with patients who received no PRP. In those patients who received intra-ovarian PRP injections there was an increase in anti-mullerian hormone (AMH) levels and antral follicle (AF) count. More importantly, there seemed to be a slightly improved live birth rate in those women who received PRP. This increase in live birth rate needs considerably more work using large numbers of patients before it can be properly confirmed or refuted. Similar studies have shown a possible benefit in using PRP to enhance endometrial thickness and embryo implantation. Whilst this is interesting initial data, it must be considered with extreme caution until it is confirmed by a clinical trial. At present, the PRP data should be viewed as experimental and most certainly not in the realms of routine fertility treatment. I would not like to see PRP added to the ever-growing list of 'add-ons'.

There is currently a lot of ongoing research into the possible use of different types of stem cells in the treatment of infertility. In my own research, I work on pluripotent (meaning that they can potentially make every tissue type in the body) very small embryonic like (VSEL) stem cells. These are found in most tissues in the body and also in PRP as described above. The interesting thing about VSEL stem cells is that they may be the 'ultimate' stem cell in the body (possibly the source of other stem cells) and they seem to be a remnant of very early embryonic development. As VSEL are in PRP then they might even be contributing to the benefits seen when PRP is used clinically. There is a considerable amount of further work needed to fully understand and use VSEL stem cells and clinical trials will be needed to prove safety and efficacy. Despite this, I believe that VSEL stem cells may have a considerable part to play in the future of regenerative medicine and they may possibly become important in the overall treatment of infertility.

Other workers have shown experimentally that spermatogonial stem cells (SSC) may be capable of restoring sperm production and fertility. In addition, there is some evidence that bone marrow derived stem cells may be capable of restoring fertility in patients suffering from diminished ovarian reserves (similar to those patients described using PRP above), poor ovarian response to medication and premature ovarian failure. A similar bone marrow stem cell approach may also be helpful in restoring the endometrium or lining of the womb.

The most important thing to say about all of these PRP and stem cell ideas is that while on the face of it, they look exciting, and something which could help many fertility patients, they are all a long, long way from being a routine treatment option in fertility clinics. Everything is in the experimental phase, not the clinical phase. If you are offered such treatment, there are a few things to remember:

- PRP and stem cell applications in fertility are not yet proven to be either safe or effective, this will only be shown be detailed clinical trial data.
- If you are offered any of these experimental treatments by a fertility clinic then assuming that you give informed consent to be part of an experimental trial, and fully understand and accept the potential risks as well as the potential benefits, then you may consider receiving such a treatment.
- If you do accept to be part of an experimental treatment study using PRP, stem cells or both, then you must not be asked to pay any amount to take part. These technologies have not yet been through clinical trial and payment for them must not be given under any circumstances.

These new ideas using PRP and stem cells are an exciting development in fertility treatment which may lead to new approaches in the future. They are of particular interest to me as I have worked in both IVF and regenerative medicine for the whole of my career. To bring these two apparently disparate specialisms together would be very satisfying for me because it would close the loop of my research over the past 40 years. Having said that, if the future clinical trial evidence shows that we were misled or even totally wrong on the interpretation of the potential benefits to patients then I would be the first person to say that the technology must not be used on fertility patients. Patient safety and clinical efficacy are the paramount considerations, without satisfying these criteria then PRP and stem cell therapy would just become another pointless expensive add-on.

Embryonic Stem Cells and Hybrids

I have written in detail over the years about embryonic stem cells, including a section in the first book of this series called The Regeneration Promise. It is beyond the scope of this book to fully discuss embryonic stem cells. I mention them simply because, for some reason, embryonic stem cells are more likely to be known about or talked about than other stem cells. This may be because of preferential treatment by the media or possibly by the fact that a picture of an embryo looks much more interesting than a picture of a stem cell. Whatever the reason it is certain that embryonic stem cells will not become part of the routine treatments offered in regenerative medicine. There may be possible treatments in the future, especially related to vision, but in general terms there are plenty of other stem cells which can do the same or even better job.

There have been some highly questionable experiments in the past related to the creation of human-animal hybrids. The concept here is to take an animal embryo, *e.g.*, a monkey, and inject it with human cells. The human cells can in theory incorporate themselves into the animal embryo and thus produce a hybrid. Such a hybrid could in theory go to term if placed into a surrogate and we could end up with monkey/human creatures. I have often failed to see the point of such experiments and they are illegal in most countries. The only thing I can really say about such experiments is that no one in their right mind should be manipulating nature at this level, no matter what the academic or financial rewards may be. There are certain things in science which are possible but should never be done and this is a classic example.

KEY POINTS OF CHAPTER 11

- The future of IVF is bright, but many changes are needed to make it a patient focussed process once again.
- Profit driven fertility services may often mean that the service provided to fertility patients is less than optimal.
- IVF is at a point of stagnation and new ideas and people are needed to 're-start' the service.
- There are several new ideas and concepts slowly entering fertility treatment but more effort and investment is needed in the development of enhanced fertility services in the future.

CHAPTER 12

A Final Thought

Peter Hollands

(Some Possible Conclusions)

No one can be a great thinker who does not recognize that as a thinker it is his first duty to follow his intellect to whatever conclusions it may lead.
John Stuart Mill

Summary: This chapter introduces the basic history of IVF and fertility treatment and sets the scene for the detailed information presented later in this book. It provides an initial overview of IVF technology from the first birth in 1978 to today and the alternatives to fertility treatment such as adoption. It also considers the growing population of Earth and the possible stagnation of fertility services.

INTRODUCTION

This book has covered many complex subjects in fertility using clear and sometimes very direct language. Thank you for sticking with it! The book has been written so that it is accessible to anyone either with just an interest in IVF and fertility treatments or to those patients who are actually currently undergoing IVF. The book has included areas of optimism, sometimes areas of great pessimism and sometimes direct criticism of the current practice of IVF. This is not to anger or directly criticise any one person or fertility clinic. The purpose of this book is to enable fertility patients to understand the process of IVF better, and to think about IVF in a critical way and not in a passive, uninvolved and accepting way. The Fertility Promise aims to empower fertility patients with the knowledge and confidence to challenge the 'status quo' to the benefit of everyone.

FERTILITY PATIENTS

Fertility patients will not change in the future. They will always be stressed, worried, frightened, optimistic, trusting, happy, unhappy and sometimes even angry. They may feel overwhelmed by forms, terminology, scans, treatments, peer pressure, family pressure, and quite often financial worries. They will all have one common target, and this is to create a family which is impossible for them without considerable technical intervention. My hope for fertility patients in the future is that the technology and delivery of fertility treatments changes such that it makes fertility treatment more reliable, affordable, accessible, understandable and effective. This will remove a lot of the stress currently piled on fertility patients and make the whole process of fertility treatment easier to cope with as a patient.

PHYSICIANS

Patrick Steptoe was the first ever physician to work in IVF and his knowledge, skill and temperament were critical in the early development of IVF. The work ethic he promoted was one of serious responsibility with the patient always being the one and only priority. He was formidable in debate, but he also listened very carefully to the opinions and ideas of others and always made evidence-based decisions. He did not suffer fools lightly and for that reason was very much trusted and respected. Patrick personally trained all of the physicians who worked in Bourn Hall Clinic in the early days, and he also gave considerable knowledge and support to nurses working on the ward and in the operating theatre.

The physicians who work in fertility today are in general terms highly professional and caring towards their patients. Nevertheless, there have been, without question, a few 'maverick' physicians since 1978. Anyone in the field will easily be able to give many examples, it is not my place to name names. These mavericks have sometimes pushed the technology and the patience of the regulatory authorities and their clinic staff to the limit and beyond. Some have even had to face legal proceedings against them as a result. Some have even won those legal cases! These maverick physicians would argue that their enthusiasm was always based around optimising patient care but in some cases the actions could be argued to be more based around personal profit and personal fame. There are several physicians who have become unjustly famous as a result of their work in IVF, some even become television personalities. This just does not feel right for a physician. Another thing which fertility physicians need to reflect on is that when they work in fertility, they are *part of a team* and not a dictating leader. This was the basic premise of Edwards, Steptoe and Purdy but there have been many physicians in fertility who have appointed themselves the self-appointed leader (and in some cases dictator) of the clinic. This is partly the blame of the medical profession in general where senior physicians, for some strange reason, may see themselves as 'above' their immediate colleagues and expect to be the one and only final decision makers. This does not work in fertility (or indeed in any area of clinical practice) and a massive medical ego (with beliefs such as 'this is my clinic, I will make the decisions') can make the lives of both staff and patients at fertility clinics a misery. I must stress that this criticism is not aimed at all physicians working in fertility, but it is a pattern of behaviour which I have experienced over the years and those who do it know full-well the damage they are doing. I have resigned once because of an intolerable physician 'running' the clinic. It was a dictatorship with a blame culture, and it was an extremely unpleasant place to work, and I believe equally unpleasant for the patients. My plea is that everyone, including physicians, need to think carefully about how they behave towards both colleagues and towards patients, to control their ego and to do more listening than talking.

CLINICAL EMBRYOLOGISTS

In the early days of IVF, Bob Edwards recruited people to work with him as Clinical Embryologists and these people were usually trusted post-graduate students from Cambridge University who had completed a PhD under his supervision. This applied to me and many of the other 'ground-breaking' Clinical Embryologists who worked at Bourn Hall Clinic in the very early days of IVF. Bob Edwards trained each one of us personally and even when he was extremely busy with international meetings, writing books and scientific publications he was always happy to 'do a shift' at the clinic. He actually always seemed happiest when he was working in the fertility laboratory. It was great to see someone who loved his work so much, he was a true inspiration and a great leader.

In those early days at Bourn Hall Clinic, a Clinical Embryologist always worked with a Laboratory Technician as an operational team for each shift which were early, day and late to cover every aspect of patient care throughout the day. The whole team of embryologists, physicians and nurses were also on call 24/7 should there be the need to carry out an egg collection out of working hours. Patient care and the service provided to patients were the absolute priority, this is sadly often not the case today. The Clinical Embryologist actually manipulated sperm, eggs and embryos and the Laboratory Technician acted in support of this by providing equipment, reagents, documentation and assistance in sterile procedures. The Laboratory Technicians generally had a first degree in science and the Clinical Embryologists usually held a Ph.D. (research degree) which was achieved in the laboratory of Bob Edwards in the Physiological Laboratory in Cambridge University. This relationship and work practice was based on that between Bob Edwards and Jean Purdy. In an academic sense Jean had the role of Research Assistant to Bob Edwards even though she was a qualified nurse and not a scientist. This Clinical Embryologist/Laboratory Technician work style was changed in the late 1980's when it became clear that it was not a cost-effective option to have two people effectively doing one job. Many of the laboratory technicians underwent extra training and became clinical embryologists in their own right.

Today, clinical embryologists have a very clear career and qualifications structure with post-graduate degrees available in Clinical Embryology and professional registration of Clinical Embryologists with organisations such as the Health and Care Professions Council (HCPC) in the UK. This ensures that safety and competence of all Clinical Embryologists.

It has sadly become a fact of life in modern IVF that clinical embryologists rarely have any role in decision making about the clinic or patient treatment. This has been taken over by physicians (who often see themselves as a 'leader' or 'owner' of the clinic) and even sometimes by totally separate management teams in very large clinics. I think that this removal of Clinical Embryologists from the management of the fertility clinic is a bad thing both for the patients and for the clinics.

FERTILITY NURSES

In the early days of IVF, the fertility nurses were general nurses who simply found working in fertility to be an interesting option to their more traditional role. They would care for female patients on the ward and also provide nursing support for procedures and patient care in the operating theatre and recovery.

Today, Fertility Nursing is a recognised specialism by the Nursing and Midwifery Council (NMC) and Fertility Nurses play a critical role in the overall care of fertility patients. The fertility patients will have the most contact of all clinic staff with the Fertility Nurses from their first appointment to their discharge at the end of treatment. Fertility Nurses provide their own consultations about the IVF process, the consents required and the self-administration of medication to the patients. These consultations are also opportunity to clarify any questions which may arise from the physician consultation. Some patients feel more comfortable to ask the Fertility Nurses questions and this should be actively encouraged in a good clinic. Fertility Nurses also carry out ultrasound scanning both for follicle growth assessment and the confirmation of a fetal heartbeat following successful IVF treatment. The Fertility Nurse is at the heart of every IVF clinic and often becomes the most trusted healthcare professionals by the fertility patients. The Fertility Nurses also provide an on-call service for patients who may have an emergency out of hours.

Today, fertility nurses are taking on more and more roles. This relies on the never-ending enthusiasm of Fertility Nurses, but it makes them vulnerable to exploitation by bosses seeking to get the same work done for less salary. Fertility Nurses can be found carrying out egg collections, giving anaesthetic and prescribing in some fertility clinics. This not only puts additional pressure onto what is already a stressful job, but it also makes the boundary between physician and nurse extremely vague. This is potentially dangerous to fertility patients and it is something which fertility clinic management should think very carefully about in the future.

CLINICS

It is the IVF clinics themselves, and the people who run them, who are at the source of the current problems in IVF. The technology (apart from rampant useless add-ons) is trying to slowly improve, and this will no doubt accelerate in the future. Clinics need to improve their communication with patients, they need to *listen* to patients and to place their patients at the centre of everything they do. This is easier said than done. The poor philosophy and bad habits in fertility clinics which have developed over the past 30 years will be difficult to change. The current workforce in IVF clinics may even find it impossible to change or have no enthusiasm at all for change. It may need the next generation of healthcare professionals working in fertility to make the changes. In the meantime, across the globe, we have thousands of fertility patients starting fertility treatment every day and the same old millstone grinds on. I would like to be optimistic that fertility clinics will change but at the same time I have a deep fear that they will not. Only time will tell.

CONCLUSION

This book has covered most aspects of fertility treatment in a style which is aimed directly at fertility patients and the general public or general reader. It has pulled no punches and has told some very hard truths, which many people may not like to see in writing. It is not my purpose to shock or to overdramatise the current problems in fertility treatment. My purpose is to educate, inform and empower fertility patients to get the very best from their complex, expensive treatment.

My own experience whilst writing this book has been very interesting. I have heard from many friends and colleagues who were very supportive and indeed asked me regularly about when it will be published. I have also heard from other people who were not quite so supportive of the idea of this book and some who were extremely negative. I am not sure what drove the negativity, but it might have been the realisation that the book might change the way they think and work. In the 40 years I have worked in, and been associated with, IVF I have seen many changes not all for the better. I have worked in many different situations from the UK to Canada and Nigeria and I have worked at many different levels from Trainee Embryologist to Scientific Director. I have worked in private clinics and in the public sector and been an academic at several Universities. The aspect which never changed was the respect and support I received from the many different patients I came across during my work. This is the global constant despite all of the problems in IVF the patients are so focussed and determined and for this they should all be commended. Fertility patients are the reason why IVF exists, and the industry should recognise this fact and begin a new era of patient focussed service.

The future of IVF is, I think, broadly good. There are many serious problems to overcome but they should not be unsurmountable with the co-operation of fertility clinics. The problem is of course that fertility clinics have got into some very bad habits and correcting or removing those bad habits will have an impact on their overall income. Sadly, IVF has become an industry and that industry, just like any other, must make profit to survive. If everything the IVF clinics offer was totally tried and tested, and the price of these services were fair and equitable with a modest profit, then I would be very happy. This is not the case at present because IVF clinics generate inflated profits and offer patients many things which are far from tried and tested. If we can move away from greed and unethical practice to prudent financial management and ethical practice then we would be well on the way to providing an excellent service for fertility patients.

Throughout this book, I have tried my best to be fair, honest and factual. If there are any areas where the reader thinks that this is not the case, then I am more than happy to enter into further discussions. Open, honest debate is always very welcome. Finally, I hope that you enjoyed this book and found it interesting, entertaining and informative. I also hope that those people working in fertility read this book and that it sparks a new level of debate and improvement which is so badly needed in IVF. I doubt that I will live to see any real change in IVF but if this book helps to get the debate and the changes started, then I will be very happy.

KEY POINTS OF CHAPTER 12

- Fertility patients are the only true constant in fertility treatment. Their aims and wishes remain the same, to have their own family.
- Fertility clinic staff would do well to reflect more on their work and their patients.
- IVF will survive in some form in the future but hopefully in a new atmosphere of honesty, integrity and professionalism.

Suggested Further Reading

A Matter of Life (1980) by Robert G. Edwards and Patrick C. Steptoe.

Life Before Birth (1989) by Robert G. Edwards.

The Regeneration Promise: The Facts Behind Stem Cell Therapies (2020) by Peter Hollands.

How to Cope with IVF: An Essential Survival Guide for First Timers (2017) by Sylvia Dunn

This is IVF and other fertility treatments: Real-life experiences of going through fertility treatments (2020) by Sheila Lamb.

IVF Got This (2020) by Collette Centeno Fox.

IVF A Detailed Guide: Everything I Wish I Had Known Before Starting My Fertility Treatments (2016) by Bianca Smith.

USEFUL WEBSITES

https://www.asrm.org/

https://www.bournhall.co.uk/

https://www.chu.cam.ac.uk/news/2019/jun/10/papers-sir-robert-edwards/

https://www.eshre.eu/

https://www.hcpc-uk.org/

https://www.hfea.gov.uk/

https://www.hfea.gov.uk/choose-a-clinic/preparing-for-your-clinic-appointment/

https://www.nhs.uk/conditions/infertility/

https://www.nhsprofessionals.nhs.uk/Campaigns/gp-bank/healthcare-assistant

https://www.nice.org.uk/guidance/conditions-and-diseases/fertility--pregnanc--and-childbirth/fertility

https://www.nmc.org.uk/

https://www.rcog.org.uk/

https://www.rcpath.org/

https://www.who.int/news-room/fact-sheets/detail/infertility

GLOSSARY

'Add-on': This is a treatment and technology which is offered with the implication that it might improve treatment cycle success rates. Add-ons are untested unproven and expensive and patients are well advised to avoid using them.

Blastocyst: This is a day 5 embryo consisting of a hollow ball of approximately 120 cells.

Cervix This is the medical term for the neck of the womb.

Cleavage Stage: This is a day 2-3 embryo where individual cells can be seen *e.g.* 2 cell, 4 cell, 8 cell.

Counsellor: This is an independent healthcare professional who is available to advise and support fertility patients. In general counsellors are grossly underused they are an excellent resource which all fertility patients should use.

Cryopreservation: This is the scientific term for freezing and it is the process use to freeze human embryos for later us.

Donor Eggs: These are eggs donated for use by fertility patients.

Donor Sperm: This is sperm donated for use by fertility patients.

Down Regulation: This is the use of medication to stop the production of all reproductive hormones. Down regulation provides the 'foundation' for ovarian stimulation to produce enough eggs for IVF.

Embryo Replacement/Transfer: This is the procedure of returning an embryo back to the patients' womb. It should be a relaxed process and the partner of the patient can also be present.

In Vitro Fertilisation (IVF): This is the process by which eggs are fertilised by sperm in the laboratory. The Latin phrase *In Vitro* translates to 'in glass' but in actual fact all of the technology used to carry out IVF is disposable clinical grade plastic and not glass.

Intracytoplasmic Sperm Injection (ICSI): This is technology which enables the embryologist to directly inject a sperm into an egg. This is particularly useful when the sperm count is low but unfortunately the technology is currently over-used in modern IVF.

Laparoscopy This is the original 'key-hole' surgery, developed by Patrick Steptoe, to collect eggs from the female patient. It requires a general anaesthetic. Laparoscopy has now been superseded by Ultrasound Guided Egg Collection.

Morula: This is a day 4 embryo consisting of tightly packed counsellorsit contains approximately 16 cells.

Oocyte: This is the egg of the female patient.

Ovarian Hyperstimulation Syndrome This occurs when the medication given to stimulate the ovaries is too high. The result is a potentially fatal complication called Ovarian Hyperstimulation Syndrome (OHSS).

Ovarian Stimulation This is the medication given to the female patient to stimulate the production of more than one egg per ovary during a treatment cycle.

Pronuclei These are two small 'blobs' seen in fertilised eggs. The pronuclei contain the DNA from the male and the female which will fuse to from a new individual.

Speculum: This is a piece of medical equipment used to open the vagina so that the cervix can be seen.

Spermatozoa These are the sperm of the male patient.

Surgical Sperm Collection: This is the collection of sperm surgically for those patients who have ongoing sperm production but produce no sperm at all in the ejaculate. It is carried out at the fertility clinic under sedation.

Trigger Injection: This is an injection (containing hCG) given approximately 36 hours before egg collection which ensures that the eggs collected will be mature and ready to be fertilised.

Two Week Wait: This is the time between embryo replacement and pregnancy test. Some patients feel the highest levels of stress during this period. If you need during the two week wait then help please contact your clinic.

Ultrasound Guided Egg Collection: This is technology which uses ultrasound to visualise the follicles in the ovary (which contain the eggs). The ultrasound is then used to guide a needle to the follicle to aspirate the fluid it contains. The egg is in this fluid and the egg can be seen by the embryologist in the laboratory using a low power microscope.

Uterus This is the medical term for the womb.

Vaginal Ultrasound Technology used to monitor follicular growth and to guide the egg collection needle.

Vitrification: This is the name given to a particular type of freezing now used for human embryos.

SUBJECT INDEX